PERFECT
SEX for Men
& for the Women Who Love Them

*How to Perfect and Enjoy Sex
for a Better Quality of Life*

*Sex and Life
Can Always Be Better*

Why Wait?

by
Chin-Ti Lin, M.D.
a certified urologist

Proctor Publications, LLC • Ann Arbor • Michigan • USA

Library of Congress Catalog Card Number: 97-68873

Publisher's Cataloging-in-Publication
(Provided by Quality Books, Inc.)

Lin, Chin-Ti
        Perfect sex for men : and for the women who love them / by
    Chin-Ti Lin. – 1st ed.
        p. cm.
        ISBN: 1-882792-51-3

        1. Sexual disorders. 2. Men—Health and hygiene. I.Title

RC875.L56 1997   616.6'9
                                        QB197-40941

Printed in the United States of America

ii

Warning – Disclaimer

This book is intended to provide a reasonable approach to sex life and its problems in men. It is solely based on current available knowledge and the experience of the author, who has been a board-certified urologist for 19 years. It is not intended as a substitute for the care of an honest caring medical professional. **The author is not legally responsible for your personal care.**

Dedication

Here is my gratitude and dedication toward all people who have supported and helped me through the path of my life thus far. They are my family, relatives, mentors, and patients.

To my parents, I do appreciate the values they passed on to me. From them, I learned to believe that; 1.) if I have to heavily rely on the medical practice to make a living, there will be a strong conflict of interest between the money-making for a living and the decision-making for patient care, and 2.) if a physician's kindness and generosity in patient care are obviously accomplished at the expense of people's money, his motives are not pure and noble enough to earn the deserved respect of the medical profession. These two values have been very important for my life and career: I have firmly guarded against them well.

To my wife, Ann, who encouraged me to write down what I have told her over the years. She has constantly supported me even at the time when the situation was not popular because of the disturbance from the prevailing sentiment with self-interest, greed, and medical hostage at stake and in the conflict among medical professionals.

To my mentors, particularly, my late chairman, Dr. Jack Lapides, I am greatly indebted to his teaching and guidance. He showed me the value of being honest in personal and professional life and the spirit of fighting for what you believed in, even while it was still not popular.

To my patients, they frequently asked me where did I obtain and learn the information and the way that I explained to them and if I have a book about it. Their repetitive inquiries urged me to write the materials that I frequently presented and discussed with them.

About the Author

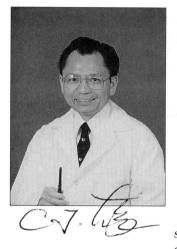

A board-certified urologist, **Chin-Ti Lin, M.D.** spent ten years in post-graduate training after medical school in 1970, including four years of training as a specialist in Urology at University of Michigan Medical Center. He has been in private practice as a urologist since 1980 and associated with University of Michigan Medical Center as a Clinical Instructor.

He has a special interest in taking care of men with sexual difficulties. Although a urologist is a surgical specialist, he approaches the issues of male sexual difficulties with common sense, low-cost, high-effectiveness, and safety. His sensible, effective approach has been proven successful for his patients and their families; he has been frequently asked, **"Where did you learn all of this? Do you have a book on this?"**

As a clinician, he wants to **help more people on a larger scale, not just one by one** at a medical office.

And at the request of his patients and their families, and to minimize the burden of the endless repetitions of sex counseling, this book was urged and written. So here is the book – **Perfect Sex for Men & the Women Who Love Them** and for you, too....

Table of Contents

- Preface .... *viii*
- My Mission as a Urologist Writer .... *xii*

Part I: General Considerations of Sex Life 1

1. Values of Sex Life 2
   - Primitive Value of Sex Life 2
   - Traditional Value of Sex Life 5
   - Contemporary Value of Sex Life
     – a Call for Justice and Respect 6

2. Social Impact of Sex Life 14
3. Recognition and Repositioning
   of the Importance of Sex Life 21

**Part II: A Brief on Anatomy and Function of
Genital Tract of Males and Females 25**

4. Origin of Sexual Organs 26
5. Structure and Function of the Penis 28
6. Comparison between Male
   and Female Sexual Organs 33

Part III: The Road to Perfect Sex 37

7. What is Perfect Sex? - Three analogies 38
8. Simplified Dynamics of Sexual Performance 47
9. Phases of the Perfect Sex Cycle 53
   - Indirect Foreplay 53
   - Direct Foreplay 56
   - Sexual Intercourse, Orgasm, and Ejaculation 57
   - Resolution and Recovery 57

10. Principles to Reach Perfect Sex 59
    - With Whom to Have Sex? 61
    - When to Have Sex? 63
    - Where to Have Sex? 65
    - A Mutual Respect for Sexual Partner &
      How to Act and Have Perfect Sex
      in Your Life 66
    - Safe Sex – a Precaution Against Sexually
      Transmitted Diseases 67

11. A Contemporary Case Study 71

12. Secrets of Obtaining a Perfect Sex Life............74
13. Artistic Views of Sex Life 81

Part IV: Sexual Difficulties in Men 85

14. Basic Requirements for
     a Good Sexual Performance..............................86
15. What are Sexual Difficulties in Men?................88
16. Erectile Difficulties as the Main Issue 91
17. Common Causes for Erectile Difficulties 96
18. Evaluation of Erectile Difficulties....................125
19. Treatment Options for
     Male Erectile Difficulties...............................138
     • Level 0: Expectant Treatment
                  (or No Treatment)..............................141
     • Level 1: Basic Sex Counseling........................142
     • Level 2: Medications by Mouth or
                  by Local Penile Injection 147
     • Level 3: Assisted Erection with Vacuum
                  Constriction Device.........................154
     • Level 4: Implantation of Penile Prosthesis –
                  the Last Resort 163

20. A Few Words on Nutrition,
     Herbs, "Accessories", and Sex 172
21. Reassessment of the Effects of Treatment 176
22. A Few Words of Caution Against Overuse
     and Abuse of Devices or Medication 178
23. Disorders of Sexual Desire (Libido)................181
24. Disorders of Ejaculation and Orgasm 183
25. A Summary of Causes and Treatment
     Options for Male Sexual Difficulties................191

Part V: A Brief on Potential Sexual Perversions 195

26. What are Abnormal Sexual Behaviors?.............196
27. What is the Social Implication of
     Abnormal Sexual Behaviors?...........................210

Part VI: Conclusion and General Advice 217

28. Conclusion on Perfect Sex 218
29. General Advice for Realistic, Safe Sex Life 221

PREFACE

While you have this book in hand, you may ask and wonder, "What is this book for? And why was this book written?" The answer is that this book's goals are **to preserve and perfect the value and beauty of sex life, to reclaim the deserved justice and respect toward sex life, to promote self-awareness and care for mens' sexual difficulties, to enhance the effectiveness of care and cooperation from, and with, medical professionals, and to help contain the cost of medical care.**

While the care for mens' sexual difficulties with a multidisciplinary approach involving the participation of specialists from urology and psychiatry and/or psychology has been traditionally promoted (especially in major medical centers) it may not be realistically available in remote, rural medical communities. And it can be very costly. Despite such an emphasis, the traditional training and practice during the period from the 1960s to the late 1980s in urology as one of surgical specialists has been oriented toward the exploration of various surgical means to rehabilitate men with erectile difficulty for their poor sexual performance. That is why urologists have been ridiculed as being penile-focused.

It has been true that many urologists tend to leave the time-consuming part of mental evaluation and management to psychiatrists or psychologists, even though much of this part of care only consists of basic sex counseling with common sense. However, such a practice has maintained a mutually appreciated, professional rapport and harmony among various sub-specialties over decades. Indeed, the colleagues of psychiatry and psychology have made a substantial contribution to the care of mens' sexual difficulties, especially for those with deeply seeded psychological disorders such as severe depression, hatred, abnormal sexual behaviors, etc.

However, in reality, surgeons mainly, and traditionally, rely on doing operations to make their living. Therefore, most surgeons and urologists love to do surgery for their professional satisfaction and financial return in order for their patients to achieve erection. This tendency of practice especially prevailed in the 1960s to the early 1990s.

Since the late 1980s, cost-containment has become a prevailing demand for medical practice. Therefore, more treatment options with less cost and invasion to achieve penile erection were continuously explored, discovered, and adapted into practice. Despite the increase in the treatment options for mens' erectile difficulties, all what many men need for their erectile difficulty, in truth, is basic sex counseling only, which is a matter of common sense.

However, for the self-interest of a trade, any trade loves, and tries hard, to keep the "knowledge" as much a secret and as tight as possible within the rein of its specialty in addition to promoting, even self-inflating, their irreplaceable importance. Doing so, the knowledge of a specialty becomes sacred and beyond the reach of the public. Such a practice is common to all professions; it is of no exception to urologists. To break the tightly guarded secrets of a specialty, I have explored the part of care that can be accomplished with common sense for mens' sexual difficulties if the patients and their sexual partners are well explained. I hope that the promotion of self-help and safety in caring and improving mens' sexual difficulties can be thereby enhanced. Meanwhile, the patients can be more knowledgeable and cooperative in order to gain more benefit from the care by medical professionals. And medical costs may decrease and be contained.

In addition, I have observed, and noted, that sex life has carried an array of endless, yet tremendous, immediate and remote impacts onto the lives of individual persons, couples, and society. In my view, **sex life is the most blessed treasured gift from God and a readily available natural resource for everyone**. Therefore, the value and beauty of sex life should be fully explored, protected, and utilized to its best.

In many sessions of counseling, the revelation of my views toward sex life and my approach to mens' sexual difficulties have easily drawn curiosity from many of my patients and their sexual partners. And they frequently asked me, "Dr. Lin, where did you learn all of this? Is there a book on this?" I usually replied, "Mr./Mrs. So and So, there is no such book around describing exactly what I just explained to you. What I just explained is nothing new at all. I merely reiterated what we humans have been doing for centuries. However, we tend to simply ignore many of the basic valuable facts of life."

Using my approach in sex counseling and care, I have observed that many men and their sexual partners were able to timely improve their undue anxiety and regain their control over sexual performance. Eventually, they rediscovered their joy of sex life, which they have missed for quite a while, months or years. Meanwhile, I quickly became confident in the way I approached many sensitive issues of sex life and its related difficulties.

Over the years I have given a number of public speeches on the related subjects of sex life to local medical professionals, women clubs, men's clubs, and local colleges. As usual, my audiences echoed and responded very positively to my approach in dealing with many sensitive issues of sex life. The positive responses from audiences, patients, and their sexual partners have reinforced my confidence in helping men with sexual difficulties, and their sexual partners, to reclaim their lost wonderland of a happy, fulfilling sex life. Naturally, as a clinician, I am eager and want to **help more people on a larger scale, not one by one at the office**. And this book was written to accomplish the goals that I have envisioned for years.

After reading this book, many men with sexual difficulties, along with their sexual partners, will regain their confidence to improve and rediscover the joy of a sex life. For the people with no sexual difficulties, they will surely gain a new way of looking at the value of sex life. Quite naturally, the joy in their sexual, personal, and social lives will be greatly enriched. For those with sexual difficulties, this book will definitely provide a practical guide to privately initiate, improve, and/or solve the secrets of their sexual difficulties timely.

In this book there is neither statistical data nor erotic graphic descriptions or pictures of real sexual acts as popularly shown, and seen, in many magazines and books. Much of the contents in this book are my views and I urge more medical professionals to do the same for the **practical benefits of the general public** because many of the professional secrets in any specialty is just a matter of common sense.

Parts I, II, and III are to serve as the foundation for perfecting sex life. Part IV is to overview the current trend of care for mens' sexual difficulties. Part V is to raise public awareness and attention to social impacts from "abnormal sexual behaviors". Finally, Part VI is to reiterate my views over the value and safety of sex life.

I hope that through your enthusiasm and efforts, the goals of this book can be accomplished to benefit you, your family, more people, society, and even the world.

Chin-Ti Lin, M.D.

My Mission as a Urologist Writer

Be Your Own Tour Guide to the Amazing Wonderland of Perfect Sex

If you don't know what and where the Wonderland of Perfect Sex is, I will show you how to find and create one, and stay there forever.

If you like to go to the Wonderland of Perfect Sex, but are still wondering, I will guide and help you go to enjoy and stay there also.

And if you are lost in the wilderness of sex life and wish to return to the Wonderland of Perfect Sex, I can help and work with you to go back there, too.

So, we can work together to rediscover and explore the beauty and value of the most blessed and treasured gift from God – Perfect Sex for our daily use, and pass them on as a special gift for our next generations.

And here I am with you.

Perfect Sex for Men

& for the Women Who Love Them

Part I

●

General
Considerations
of Sex Life

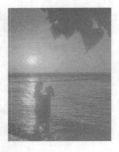

To live up to the value that a person believes in and trusts is the motivation for how a person would behave in life.

Values of Sex Life

1

While the activities of sex life comprise a major part of peoples' lives, its contents have evolved dramatically since ancient times to reflect and meet the present and practical need for individual survival and human existence. Therefore, it would be interesting and worthwhile to overview what has been going on in sex life over time.

To reveal the changes of the value of sex life over time, let us view it in three historical phases – **primitive, traditional, and contemporary value.**

Primitive Value of Sex Life

Both plants and animals have to use some form of sexual behavior to make the chromosomes from both sexes join together in order to assure the continuation of their own species. And as you know, plants cannot have direct contacts, like animals do, to put genetic characters from both sexes together in order to produce their next generation of plant life. However, the power of Nature makes the task of continuing their species possible. Well known to us, some plants rely on wind or water to bring the characters of both sexes together; for other species of plants, insects and birds have done a good job for them.

In the animal world, an active and direct contact of genital organs of both sexes is required to complete the process of bringing the chromosomes of both sexes together. This act is known as *copulation*. The process of copulation is somewhat different from species to species, depending upon their class in the animal kingdom. For animals in the lower classes, this process is not easily visible to all of us because of their tiny body size. Quite often, they can only be seen under a microscope. Therefore, the observation of copulation of the animals in lower classes has been the privileges of scientists or of students studying them.

For higher classes of animals, the behaviors of copulation have been frequently observed by almost all of us because their body sizes are large enough and therefore obviously visible. Some common examples of domestic animals are chickens, cats, dogs, cows, etc. If you have ever lived in the countryside on a farm, most of you will have plenty of opportunities to see how domestic animals behave sexually. The sexual scenes of copulation, quite frequently, attract the curiosity of many youngsters who will stare at them and come back to ask their parents many questions about these animals.

For animals in the wild such as tigers, lions, deer, raccoons, baboons, monkeys, chimpanzees, and even humans, their sexual behaviors have been well observed and documented through the dedicated efforts of many scientists who study them. The very detailed scenes of sexual behaviors have also been shown in many documentary movies such as those on the Discovery Channel or the Public Broadcasting System. The sexual behavior to produce the next generation in these animals is more commonly called *sexual intercourse*, although, in essence, it is a form of copulation.

In general, their intercourse results in producing next generations. It is completed through their mutual agreement and only after a period of gaming pursuit for such an ultimate sexual act. However, their pursuit for sexual intercourse only occurs at certain time of the year in their lives. Other than this certain time of the year, they are just not interested in sex at all. Instead, they are largely interested only in resting and playing so they can sharpen their skills of self-defense and find food for survival. However, when their mating season comes, the effects of their sexual hormones will make them disinterested in almost anything but sex. At such times, they will behave very differently. We call this being in *Estrus*, or *heat*. Domestically, you may have heard and seen female cats while they are in heat meowing all day and night to attract male cats to have intercourse with them. A similar phenomenon has been well known for dogs and even cows. An extreme example of this mating frenzy (heat) was observed in a female baboon having as many as 23 unions of sexual intercourse with 3 different males over a period of 10 hours.

Then, how is the sex life in humans? Humans have done the same as well. However, it is distinctively different to observe that sexual intercourse does not take place only at the certain times of life, or the year. Instead, both males and females pursue the opportunities to have sexual intercourse as a part of their daily lives over a very long life span. Clearly, the goal of sex life has exceeded its original intuitive purpose for procreation. Obviously it carries a strong intentional desire for pleasure as a part of life.

Therefore, in a primitive sense, we can firmly state that the most primitive value of sex life is for procreation. Procreation has made all the species of the biological world able to compete for existence and to allow their progressive evolution to take place. For human beings, the same rule applies.

Traditional Value of Sex Life

What is the traditional value of sex life in human history? To answer this seemingly simple question, we need to look into what has happened in human history with a focus on sex life. Theoretically, throughout history, all the combined human mental and physical activities in the past have exerted their own effects on our expression of sexual behaviors today. Unfortunately, not all materials in history are considered "accurate" or "accountable". In reality, the information that we can count on today is traceable only in the available records. For this, let us review what we humans have performed in the sexual aspect of life from "traceable" history.

In ancient times, either in the West or East, most of the records about sex were described as a myth of nature. And as you might have read, there have been a lot of stories describing the origin and power of human sex affairs. For example, in the West, ancient Greeks compared the power of sexual affairs to a force that coordinates the whole universe and that sexual desires provide an ultimate gravitational force to pull all the matters of human life together. To this fact, many interesting lovely stories were written by Greeks and Romans about a handsome but mischievous boy, Eros, or sometimes called Cupid.

As to the origin of sex, a lovely story about Hermaphrodite, a strange creature of one body with two faces, two arms, and two legs, was created and passed on over centuries. This strange creature was then split into two parts by God because God was outrageously jealous about Hermaphrodite's original self-sufficient sexual function.

In the East, by ancient Chinese, the power of sex in the male and female was thought to be the ultimate force of nature to keep every thing in the universe in harmony and balance. It is so-called Yin-Yang.

However, in the real life of humans, the power of sex has unfortunately been exploited for centuries by gender, churches, and ruling groups for self-serving purposes of dominance, control, and selfishness. As a result, males have been in a more active and dominant position as compared to females who have been more passive and subordinate.

Clearly, in a traditional sense, sexual activities have been mainly for procreation and for the self-serving control and pleasure of males over females.

Contemporary Value of Sex Life
– A Call for Justice and Respect

The traditional value of sex life has taken its route from ancient times up until the period of the last three centuries.

During this time, through influences and concepts of science, the Industrial Revolution (1760) took place and pushed forward the social structure and the flow of thinking about the social value of sex life. Gradually, for the purpose of mutual and efficient survival, the position and balance of the value of sex life has also undergone a fast pace of change. As a result, the power of dominance and control by males over females has slowly weakened. To explore, and understand the motives for pursuing sexual pleasure, Sigmund Freud (1856-1939) was credited as one of the first to explore the territory of sex and its value. He believed that sexual erotic attraction was the centrifugal force of all affectionate human relationships. Many of his thoughts have directly and indirectly influenced many other later thinkers about the value of sex life today. As the new territory of reassessing the value of sex life was being explored, the pressure for change was building and rising. From the 1950s, the movement of womens' liberation started to emerge and evolve. The need for fairness to share the instinctive and intentional roles of sex life between males and females was becoming self-evident, in spite of the presence of some sporadic resistance here and there. The works of many subsequent philosophers, psychologist, and women activists have further contributed to the momentum to materialize the identifiable need for fairness in many aspects of sex life. Therefore, where are we and in which direction should we steer the new value of sex life? With a little bit of common sense, we will humbly realize the direction we should be moving along. For further consolidating and benefiting our attained value of sex life through a long historical struggle, we need to find ways to make the best use of all the potential beneficial effects of sex life for us now and for the generations to come.

Although a great progress in equalizing rights and fairness for males and females has been made over the last century, the traditional value of the female sexual role being solely for procreation is still deeply embedded in the minds of many males and females. Today, many females are still intimidated and discouraged from pursuing and exploring the real essence of their sexual activities in life. Despite this, the direction and flow of the female's sexual role has never been so revealing as it is today. Most of us would agree that males and females are equally responsible for the contribution and control over mental, physical, spiritual, and materialistic activities in spite of their biological difference. The acceptance of this concept should be the basic foundation to appreciate the contemporary value of sex life. Therefore, males and females should equally share the opportunity to contribute and receive the joy of sex life under terms of cooperation and mutual respect.

What is the real force that made such a history? Simply put, it is the presence of the dual purposes of sex life in humans; **the instinctive act for procreation and the intentional desire for pleasure.** Consequently, there have been many sexual ramifications in personal and social levels. Although, in a primitive sense, the biological instinctive acts of Nature makes both sexes copulate for procreation, sexual pleasure is an attraction which may be a part of intense momentary compensation that induces males and females to participate in the activity of reproduction. Such an attraction may make the participants "addicted" and urge males and females to constantly pursue sexual pleasure by any means. On social levels, such urges and addictions have led to many social activities to take place and evolve throughout history. Unfortunately, while the position of this intentional driving force for sexual pleasure is out of place and balance, sexual violence such as rapes or sexual harassment will take place.

On a personal level, we realize the fact that human beings are free from estrus (or heat) of animals. Instead, our sexual behaviors first originate from the feeling of what we see, hear, think, and imagine, and secondly, a subsequent desire to pursue acts. In general, the actions are intentionally directed to make us feel satisfied and fulfilled inside as well as outside. However, the outcome of intended actions may be a success or a failure. A success in acts will favorably produce a positive reward of complex emotions. Conversely, a failure in acts will unfavorably bring in a complex of negative emotions. All the experience in perceiving negative and positive memories and emotions will be retained in our minds on conscious or subconscious levels. These experiences will have a very far-reaching effect on a person's personality and the health of an overall sex life in the future. The positive memories may include all the rewarding emotions such as pleasure, joy, love, hope, realistic pride, and fulfillment for ourselves and for our sexual partners. Those of a negative nature may be the feelings of uncertainty, frustration, anxiety, shame, guilt, and even anger. The intensity of a desire to act and the nature of the acts are usually proportionally related to the recollection of prior positive or negative emotional complexes. Our ability to direct and transform intentional sexual desire without estrus (or heat) into sexual acts has made sex life among humans much different and more complicated with all the memories and emotions just described.

The experience of learning, maturing, and mastering the

ability to handle all the negative and positive emotions from birth to "independent" adulthood is a very intense and perplexing job. Also, the importance of its impact on any future behavioral expressions of sex life and general personality is very obvious.

After realizing the generally expected progression from thoughts (sexual desires, or urges) to actions (sexual behaviors) in human life, let us look hard into what really happens to a person in the family and society.

A sex life does not just begin in adulthood. It starts its journey from the very beginning and continues to the very end of life on subconscious and conscious levels. In infancy, sexuality is largely influenced by the quality of all kinds of physical contacts, pleasurable and trustworthy, or unpleasant and dangerous. To demonstrate this effect on sexuality, it has been shown that infants who receive good mothering masturbate by one year of age and those who are poorly mothered do not. Although during this period an instinctive response is more predominant as compared to intentional responses, this observation strongly suggests there is a significant effect on sexual response from their interaction with surroundings. Meanwhile, infants learn the sense of being male or female. In short, during this period, through instinctive responses, they gain trust and enjoyment of physical closeness as well as the ability to form healthy and loving bonds. This example is to remind us as parents and adults to **never overlook the importance of interaction with children around, even while they are at a very young age.**

Throughout life, a person learns much of the intentional value and significance of sex life from his surroundings. One constantly adjusts and adapts to different forms of expression of sexual behaviors at different stages of life. The goal of one's active, delicate, lifelong learning is to **first meet the need to pursue social approval** and **secondly, to satisfy the desires of sexual pleasure.** One then becomes able to apply the ideas of when, where, with whom, and how to show what forms, or degrees, of one's sexual behavioral expression in order to conform with the standards of both one's family and society.

In short, learning an appropriate pattern of sexual expression in early life is very important. It will eventually show up and affect one's sexual behaviors in adulthood. Understandably, in addition to the inborn and instinctive ability to sense and act sexually, children first sense what their parents do with an increasing degree of intention. In time, children expand their scope of ability to express the sexual behaviors that are appropriate within the family. As age increases, the factors affecting what one learns will gradually expand beyond the limit of direct parental supervision. The child then starts to learn from whatever he can see, hear, smell, and touch from all the directions in his surroundings outside the home. Of course, the standards of social approval and personal sexual satisfaction can vary widely because of the difference in racial, cultural, geographic, economical, religious and political backgrounds.

To assist young people to go through and develop such a complicated transition, **all adults in society should take a share in the responsibility as a role model.** At home, parents should be the initial model of human sexuality of adulthood. **A natural and proportional revelation of sexual behaviors in daily life is surely healthy for a good relationship of a couple as well as a role model for their children.**

The practice of sex life surely guarantees a society that generations will continue, although infertility for various reasons does happen to some unfortunate couples. This fact has helped sex life to earn its deserved respect. However, even today, in some religious teachings and preaching, a sex life is considered solely for procreation. To an extreme, even a thought of sex might be considered to be shameful and sinful in some families and religions. The temptation and discipline to preach this belief are still prevailing in many situations and places. However, in spite of these intended efforts, the contents of our daily sex life have undergone unlimited changes and expansions over time because of the inevitable intentional urge to pursue sexual pleasure. It has been especially obvious over the last thirty years. Now, the ever-expanding expression of promiscuity through sexual behaviors has brought significant threats to our lives with sexually related diseases such as gonorrhea, syphilis, AIDS, etc., and increasing social disorders with violence such as sexual harassment and rapes.

The progression of these threats has been seemingly unstoppable, although we have been making more and more efforts in sexual education in private and public sectors, and generating ever increasing rules, regulations, and laws to curb and contain them.

Apparently, the joy of sex is no longer the privilege of married couples as adopted in many cultures for centuries. **The discipline, limitation, and restriction of sexual behaviors do not effectively stop or contain the urgent power of pursuing the joy of sex. This is a reality.** Could something be done to minimize and even eliminate the risks from overwhelming variations in sexual behaviors? For the sake of having a long enduring effect, it is of no doubt in my mind, and most people will agree, that **education with an emphasis on personal responsibility is the key impor-**

tance to all needed efforts. If we just teach and impress upon our children that the joy of sex life is only for adults and that they have to wait their turn until they reach their adulthood, will they listen to what we adults say to them? History has told us that it is not possible, and it is impractical to believe this way.

But in spite of the complexity of views of the practice of sex life, let us take a realistic look and examine the contents of sex life in today's social life.

The pressure to pursue the joys of sex, by young or old, is enormous and overwhelming. We cannot just stop it. However, we can divert it for the benefit of life. In my view, the joy of sex life is **a great and wonderful blessing, a gift from God that allows humans to have a special form of recreation or mini-vacation in their daily life.** After a day of dedication and hard work for yourselves, family and society, don't you deserve such a blessed treatment with the joy of sex. Such a blessed intimacy will further nourish a closer relationship with your sexual partner and a more adventurous life to come.

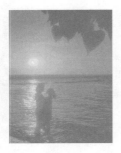

Every act has its immediate and ripple effects on the originator and its surroundings. Sex life is especially obvious and true; but although it is your right to enjoy, it is also your obligation to be the role model for following generations.

2
Social Impact of Sex Life

What is the impact of sex life upon our modern society? From the earliest beginnings of humanity, and throughout all recorded human history, there remain two desires that have an enormous social impact upon society: the desire for food, and the desire for sex. As the ancient Chinese philosopher Confucius (551 BC - 479 BC) stated thousands of years ago, **"Food and sex are the nature of life."** In America, this is especially true and noticeable because of the media. There is a continuous bombardment of commercials that promote diet, weight loss programs, self-help books for obesity, etc. And at the same time, Americans are receiving a barrage of sexual innuendos from many advertisements, television programs, movies, music, etc. While the social effects for food are easily understandable, we need to examine the socially related matters resulting from human sexuality in a more detailed manner.

What is the direct impact that sex life has upon a society? First of all, there are too many to list. While many effects are subtle, others are very obvious and immediate. And to illustrate the obvious direct effects, let us examine the following questions:

1. *Do you believe that a person will be happier in her/his daily living if she/he is satisfied with their sex life?*

2. *Do you believe that the atmosphere of a family tends to be happier if a couple living together are satisfied with their sex life? And the children being raised under that happier atmosphere, will they also be healthier and happier?*

3. *Do you believe that a society will be happier and live better if more people and families are filled with a happier and more satisfied sex life?*

I have frequently asked these three questions of my audience whenever I have given speeches on the subject of **"The Social Impact of Sex Life Upon Society and Life."** With no exception, the audience nodded their heads to say "Yes" to these questions. Apparently, the audience endorsed and agreed with these three important issues. All people want to have a successful and fulfilling sex life that will allow them to live, work, and raise children in a happier atmosphere. It is obvious that a good sex life will generate an immediate effect in our daily lives.

No further words are needed to stress the importance, the value, and the power of a happy fulfilling sex life.

However, about fifty percent of marriages end up in divorce. Why is this? Because they are not happy living together. The value and beauty of being married and living together has tarnished. While many issues may appear to cause couples to break up, the single most important reason is usually a poor sex life. But many of them did not recognize their sexual inadequacies and problems that caused their separation. And quite often, they even rejected the thought, idea, or even the mention of a poor sexual relationship. People like this are in denial.

From the earliest colonial days until present, sexual evolution and revolution has taken place in America and it continues with each new generation. From the earliest times of strict Puritan standards in America to the present age of single-parent families, one thing remains the same; the birth of a baby is the direct result of sexual intercourse (except for artificial fertilization). Everyday, there are announcements of marriages and birth of babies to couples. For either occasion, we congratulate the couple on their marriage or the birth of their child. This becomes the "happy time" of life – celebrating the joys of mating and the happiness of giving birth to a new life.

What was the single most important reason for any couple to get married? Love! Love has been the number one reason mentioned. When couples want to get married, they firmly state that they really love one another and they are willing to do anything for each other during the "good times" and the "bad times" of their lives. Therefore, they get married. However, there also comes a time for some couples to separate because they no longer are willing to live under the same roof and/or sleep on the same bed. And unfortunately, there are announcements of divorces in local newspapers, sometimes mentioning friends and relatives as well. It is interesting, but sad, to note that in our society, the number of people filing for a divorce and/or filing to get married are almost equal (according to a monthly credit bureau report).

When couples separate and/or divorce, what happens to the life they shared together? How drastic and sarcastic is the comparison between the vows that couples exchange at their wedding ceremony and the unhappiness and dissatisfaction that is revealed at the time of their separation. This is the "unhappy time" of life. What happened to the love they perceived and created for their marriage vows? While couples are falling in love, they demand a lot of attention of each other. They want to be with each other all the time, talk to one another all the time, and are in varying degrees of physical contact when they are together. Unfortunately, after marriage, many of these daily rituals seem to fade away. In other words, they are no longer making an effort to maintain or sustain their close and intimate relationship. Love without a true determination for sacrifice is deceiving and not real. To reverse such a tragedy in marriage, care and love for one another should be continuously expressed in daily living, not simply on special occasions such as a birthday or an anniversary.

To show an analogy of a human relationship, many of you have observed how healthy a house plant will grow when it is given proper nourishment, water, light, and all of its needs are met in a timely fashion. Likewise, the treatment for a happy and healthy relationship also takes proper nourishment and care, but is extremely more complicated than that of a plant. However, the general principle applies.

No matter what the reasons are for couples to live together, there is one thing in common; they have most likely practiced "sex" on a regular basis in some form or another. In reality, we do know that many couples become married because of unwanted pregnancies. In addition, many couples live together simply for fun and/or companionship, or to break away from a family situation. In general, the afore-mentioned conditions are more likely to be less bonding and therefore temporary.

Unfortunately, some married couples are not satisfied with their sex lives, and consequently, their sexual dissatis-faction may eventually lead to a divorce. But before their divorce proceeding, there is a time to resolve their problems with all available remedies, but they may never mention, or even face, the issue of sexual dissatisfaction. Why? It is not because they do not want to talk about it. Instead, they are too shy, too ashamed, or they simply hate one another too much to talk about it. Or they just don't know how to find the help they so desperately need.

Who or what makes people avoid meaningful discus-sions of sex when their sex lives are in trouble and possibly becoming the main reason for their marital problem? There is little doubt that traditions, morals, religious beliefs, family upbringing, and/or societal pressures have taught many people to behave in such a way as not to trust "open discus-sions" or "private discussions" that concern intimate sexual matters. This is truly unfortunate, for the road to "healing" is paved with "trust" and "open discussion". When people share their true feelings and emotions with someone they care about, they are revealing to the other person that they trust and love them enough to expose their innermost feelings. Being "vulnerable" can have its drawbacks – and its rewards. The downside of "personal vulnerability" is that the other person will trivialize the situation and not be serious. But the rewards for "personal vulnerability" are numerous. The "receiver" sees and immediately understands your personal and true feelings. Everything is revealed and is in the open. You are telling the other person that you care enough about them to want a resolution of the problem and that you are willing to do anything to accomplish that goal. Therefore, do not avoid any meaningful discussion of sex when your sex life is possibly causing marital problems. Remember, running away from, or avoiding, problems never resolves or solves anything. **And in order for a couple to experience "perfect sex" in their relationship, "communication and trust" must always be a two-way street that is frequently traveled.**

Therefore, when we ask the following question; "What is the social impact, or 'ripple' effect, of a satisfying sex life upon society?" We must look at all aspects of the answer, directly and indirectly. When both people in a loving relationship are sexually satisfied, the outward manifestation of positive results may be seen in all aspects of their lives, financially, professionally, and economically. Sexual satisfaction allows a person to develop a deep concern about one's welfare and prosperity in everyday life. A person is willing and able to work harder and longer because they are able to concentrate better. And as a person becomes more efficient in their career, they tend to grow and prosper in their profession. And when there is growth in a person's profession, there will be greater financial rewards. All aspects of society seem to benefit from the "ripple effects" of an individual's satisfying sex life. It becomes visibly evident in the person, at home, and even in the workplace.

If a man is satisfied with his sex life, the fact implies that he possesses good skills in communication, which he can use no matter where he goès, and that he would be happier in his daily living. With his good skills and happier attitude, he will be able to learn faster and deal with his surroundings more effectively. As a result, it is easier for him to stand out and promote himself. Consequently, he will be more able to make more money. While he is able to make more money, he would naturally spend more in dining, clothes, travelling, and many other activities.

Obviously, a satisfied fulfilling sex life can produce an endless, positive, constructive chain of events which will stimulate and improve all aspects of personal, professional financial, and economic life.

In contrast, a dissatisfied, unfulfilling sex life can generate an endless negative, destructive chain of events which will diminish and impair all aspects of a person's life. The details of all the negativities are within anyone's imagination.

G reed and predominance have led to abuse and misuse in sex life. It is the time to restore its graciousness, beauty, and respect.

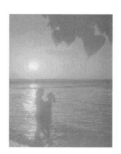

3

Recognition and Repositioning of the Importance of Sex Life

Up to this point, it is clear that there are no words sufficient enough to describe the power, importance, value, and beauty of a good sex life. However, today, what are people's common response or reaction to the issue of sex life? In general, they are in a negative tone, being shy, shamed, sinful, guilt, fearful, afraid, upset, angry, offending, and humiliating, although in recent years the trend of reaction to the issues of sex life has become somewhat more favorable, supportive, and friendly. Nonetheless, a struggle to pursue a satisfactory, fulfilling sex life continues among many people. And the rate of divorces, unwanted pregnancies, single-parent families, teen pregnancies, rapes, domestic violence, etc. is still at their alarming height. These facts strongly present the bottom line of the handicap in many unsolved issues of sex life. Despite these realistic difficulties in sex life, many people even still pretend that they did not hear it and would intentionally not touch the issues related to sex life at all.

Why? Is there a barrier to, or a phobia of, sexual issues? I hope not. Historically, indeed, the value and respect of sex life has been distorted for selfish reasons by many self-interest groups. Then, people have deliberately misused and even abused sex life at the expense of someone's sufferings. However, we know that a satisfactory, fulfilling sex life has its own merits of tremendous power, importance, value, and beauty for every person, every couple, and every society to use constructively. Why can't people change the direction of thinking and practice in sex life from the camp of negativity to a positive one and let the power, importance, value, and beauty of sex life out of the closet to work for us?

To accomplish this goal, undoubtedly, humans need to take action. And now is the best time for people to courageously recognize our unfortunate mismanagement of sex life in the past and move in the right direction of thinking and practice to promote the value and beauty of a good sex life for our good use.

Can we do it? Of course, we can. First, as usual, we need to have the courage to admit the "historical mistakes" of mistreating sex life. Second, we need to appreciate the equal importance of all aspects of sex life. Third, let's just do it. How? I have my proposal to share with you. Please read on. We can make it happen.

Although the traditional dominance and control by males over females have distorted the true value of sex life, a filtration of available historical facts should help us return to a reasonable path and a better outlook to harmonize our lives by perfecting our sex lives.

Now, as explored and discussed above, the importance of the true value of sex life for a person, a couple, and/or a society is so self-revealing that it deserves a new look – and respect. Unfortunately, it has still been misplaced in its traditionally suppressed position. Now is the proper time to reposition its deserved value in a more prominent and gracious spot in our daily lives so that everyone's sex life will receive more loving, tender care. We then need to handle it in a more positive, constructive, open, and gracious manner. Naturally, it will radiate its inherent power to benefit all the people of society.

Eventually, we can take advantage of its value and make the best use of its beneficial effect for our sexual partners, society, and ourselves. Don't you like this idea? The next step to fulfill the dream of changing your concept of sex life is your *REAL ACTIONS* to bring the truth of sex life into your daily living. Good luck! God blesses you!

Part II

●

A Brief on Anatomy and Function of Genital Tracts of Males and Females

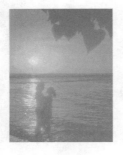

A ny organ has its origin and specific use; it is divine for a good use, not for misuse or abuse.

Origin of Genital Organs of Males and Females

4

The detailed and progressive evolutionary changes of forming the genital organs of both males and females are well beyond the scope of this book. However, a brief discussion of the genitalia is necessary for most people to better understand sexual performance, difficulty, and treatment.

After a sperm from the father and an egg from the mother unite through sexual intercourse, the fertilized egg starts its rapid, repetitive process of cell splitting (division) from one cell to two, to four, then to eight, and to all the cells of the whole body under a strict guidance of pre-programmed instructions from both parents' chromosomes and genes. This scenario is the most common one, although occasionally, more than one egg and/or artificial insemination may be involved for reproduction.

The formation of a male or female child is under the close guidance of so-called sex chromosomes. In males, they are XY chromosomes, in females, XX chromosomes. Inside this paired chromosomes are numerous and precise messages for the fertilized egg to follow and divide in the direction of forming a boy or a girl. Essentially, and eventually, the genital organs, either internal or external, will be entirely different in their structures (gross anatomy) and functions. Up to about the 50th day of pregnancy inside the womb of mothers, the shape of the genital organs is actually about the same.

From that time on, as the body further develops, male and female genital organs take their shapes to form those for males or females under the influences of various hormonal activities. Near the end of the term of pregnancy, you see the distinct and different pictures of external genital organs of males and females about 98% of the time. For more details, if you are really interested, you may review some books on this subject; human embryology.

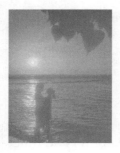

*K*nowing the structure and function of an organ with compassion will make it work better for you.

Structure and Function of the Penis

5

Structure of the Penis

The penis is composed of three cylinder-like structures as illustrated in Figure 1 on the next page. The paired two are together called *corpora cavernosa* and are solely responsible for penile erection. They lie side by side in the dorsal aspect of the penis for three-quarters of their length, which you see as the pendulous (hanging) part of the penis. Their proximal quarter is separate and attached to the under surface of the inferior part of the pubic bone, called *ischiopubic rami*, which you cannot see. And a single one right below the juncture of the paired corpora cavernosa encloses the *urethra*, the channel to allow urine to pass from the bladder, and contributes only partially to an erection.

Figure 1

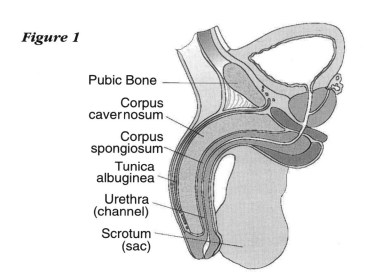

Pubic Bone

Corpus cavernosum

Corpus spongiosum

Tunica albuginea

Urethra (channel)

Scrotum (sac)

Each cylinder is surrounded by a sheath of dense and thick tissue, which is the toughest part of the body, called *tunica albuginea*. (Figure 2 next page). In addition, these three cylinders are encased by a less dense layer of tissue, called *Buck's fascia*. Under a microscope, the inside of each cylinder shows that the structure of the tissue is like a sponge, inside of which consists of smooth muscles. Among the smooth muscles are innumerous spaces for free communication, and for accepting and holding, the needed blood for an erection while the message of mental and physical stimulation is transmitted to these muscles through the nerve system to the penis.

Blood Supply to the Penis (Figure 2)

Blood supply to the penis comes from two, end arteries, one on each side of the internal pudendal artery, which originates from the internal iliac artery and supplies blood

Figure 2

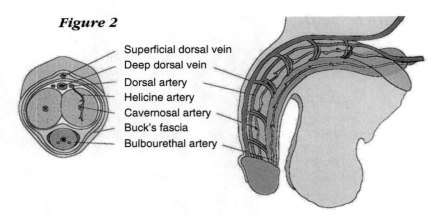

Superficial dorsal vein
Deep dorsal vein
Dorsal artery
Helicine artery
Cavernosal artery
Buck's fascia
Bulbourethal artery

to the pelvic organs. Under normal healthy condition, mental and/or physical stimulation will send the signals of sexual stimulation to the brain.

After these signals pass through an internal managing process in a special part of the brain, another signal returns from the brain to dilate the blood vessels that feed the penis and subsequently the smooth muscles that lie inside the sponge bodies. This increase in blood flow to the penis will fill up the spaces among the sponge-like tissue. And the filling up of the spaces inside sponge bodies stretches the veins inside the sheath of sponge bodies in a "shearing" direction in order to partially block the blood flow out of the penis. This phenomenon dramatically increases the pressure inside the cylinders and an erection can be initiated, maintained, and sustained. However, there is occasionally a defect of the veins inside the sheath of the cylinder structures from which these veins cannot be blocked effectively by the shearing and stretching action as just described. As a result, an erection can not be maintained. The deficiency or blockage of the arteries and veins of the penis will be further discussed in Part IV.

Nerve Supply to the Penis (Figure 3)

The penis gets its nerve supply from both autonomic (parasympathetic and sympathetic) and somatic (sensory and motor) nerves. The parasympathetic nerve fibers come out of the second, third and fourth sacral spinal cord segments and the sympathetic nerve fibers arise from the eleventh thoracic to the second lumbar spinal cord segments. The ultimate ability of these two types of nerve fibers can cause the smooth muscles of the blood vessels and sponge bodies inside the penis to relax, or contract, and produce either the erection or the flaccidity of the penis. The nerve fibers that sense touch for the penis originate from the sensory receptors in the skin and the head (glans) of the penis and eventually go into the second to fourth sacral nerves.

Figure 3

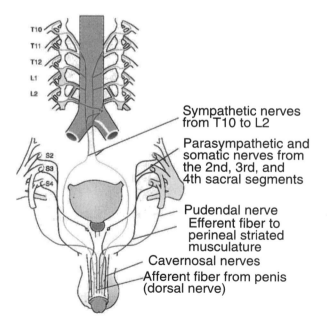

Sympathetic nerves from T10 to L2

Parasympathetic and somatic nerves from the 2nd, 3rd, and 4th sacral segments

Pudendal nerve Efferent fiber to perineal striated musculature

Cavernosal nerves

Afferent fiber from penis (dorsal nerve)

Mechanism of Erection

Mental sexual stimulation itself alone (central or psychogenic) or physical stimulation to the penis (peripheral or reflexogenic), or a combination of both can initiate a series of complicated biochemical reactions from which an endproduct, called cGMP, is produced inside the penis. This cGMP is the ultimate substance to relax smooth muscles and, therefore, initiate the process of developing an erection. Meanwhile, cGMP is then degraded by the activity of an enzyme called *phosphodiesterase* (PDE). There are at least six types of PDEs in the human body; the PDE types 2, 3, 4, and 5 are found inside the penis. The type 5 PDE is the predominant one inside the sponge bodies of the penis. Blocking the effect of this PDE type 5 can therefore increase the amount of cGMP and subsequently intensify the relaxation of the smooth muscles of sponge bodies and blood vessels to the penis and therefore produce a more rigid erection. *Sildenafil* (Viagra) has such a blocking ability. That is how this new drug works for improving penile erections. (see page 148 - 150).

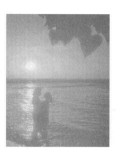

***R**ealizing the difference with respect can make a difference in passion.*

6

Comparison of Male and Female Genital Organs

We all recognize that the appearance of male and female genital organs is clearly different; however, each sexual organ of the male and of the female comes correspondingly from the same primitive tissue. For example, the sac (scrotum) of males and the lips (labias) of the vagina in females originate from the same primitive tissue and are similar in appearance during the early stage of pregnancy. But at birth their appearance is obviously different. Also, the head of the penis in males and the clitoris in females, and the testicles of males and the ovaries of females are the paired resemblance between males and females.

However, despite the difference in their appearance, these corresponding parts of sexual organs have the same source of blood and nerve supply and control. Therefore, imaginably and understandably, a damage or impairment to the tissue, blood, and nerve of the paired organs will produce similar adverse effects in the response to sexual stimulation for both males and females.

In reality, the focus of the issue on sexual difficulties in men has been the matter of erection, the cause of which will be discussed in the following section.

The detail of female sexuality is well beyond the intended scope of this book. For interested parties, please refer to other related books for more details.

Important Aspects of Male Genital Organs for Action and Treatment

After being aware of the overall and microscopic structures, and the blood and nerve supply of the penis, and understanding the differences, as well as the similarities, in the genital organs of males and females, it will be easier to understand why in some circumstances a penile erection cannot be initiated, maintained, or sustained.

As just previously described, certain parts of male and female genital organs are transformed from the same origin of primitive tissue during gestation; therefore, the origins of circulation (blood supply) and innervation (nerve supply) of certain corresponding parts of male and female genital organs are the same. However, they carry different names. For example, the head of the penis (glans penis) and the sac (scrotum) of males have the same origin of nerve and blood supplies as the clitoris and the lips of the vagina in the females. These areas are the primary sensitive areas to receive the signals of physical stimulation and to initiate instinctive and arousing effects. That is why, in these areas, both males and females masturbate themselves through proper mental and physical stimulation, especially the head of the penis in males and the clitoris in females. Both the penis and the clitoris will become hard and erected under proper stimulation; although, as you know, the erection of the penis develops faster and is really more obvious than that of the clitoris in females.

In order to achieve an erection, the nerves and muscles of these organs have to coordinate perfectly in their working conditions and sequences. Through their uninterrupted and seamless coordination, a sufficient amount of blood will increasingly flow to these organs and maintain a balanced high pressure inside their sponge tissue. An erection can then be developed, maintained, and sustained for sexual intercourse. **Therefore, any damage to the nerves, muscles or blood supply of the penis, or any combination of these three, can gradually or suddenly change the ability of initiating, maintaining, or sustaining an erection**. For men, they become impotent because of poor, or no, erection. For females, it is less a problem because vaginal penetration is still possible without an erected clitoris. That is why no, or poor, erection (erectile difficulty) has been the key concern of the issue in male sexuality. In spite of this obvious and visible difference, it is by no means that the sexual difficulties in women have been less a problem or deserve less concern. This understanding is especially important for men to know, and recognize, in order to perfect their sex lives.

Part III
●
The Road to Perfect Sex

There is always a road to reach a goal. The road to perfect sex has been inside and within the reach of any human being. Unfortunately, it has been ignored and ruined. It is the time to rediscover it and put it into its best use forever.

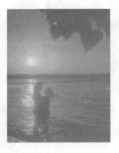

Perfecting is the core spirit of art and sex life because at its best, sex life is an art.

What is Perfect Sex?
– Three Analogies

7

The answer to this question is simple: Nothing is perfect. So there is always some room for improvement. That is why we must concentrate on the "pursuit" of perfection, rather than "focusing" on being perfect at something.

To many people, "perfection" is a word of high emotion and expectation. Simply put, this word expresses a mental state of their complete satisfactions with what they see, feel, sense, and create. The degree of being "perfect" in any event varies from time to time, place to place, and from person to person, and sometimes, even for the very same person. In other words, one's idea of being "perfect" may not be another's idea of being "perfect".

To be perfect is not easy, not to mention impossible. But in everyday life, it is not uncommon to note that there are times when you don't even get along well with yourself. Understandably, to live in a perfect harmony with yourself would be a monumental task. And to live in a perfect harmony with another person means that you would have to understand, respect, and be aware of his/her "wants and needs" all of the time; which, in reality, would be an impossibility. Therefore, to live with someone and share your life with him/her, is to realize that your "degree of perfection" may have to be significantly adjusted and increased. You have to provide for the needs of two people, your sexual partner and yourself; and this is only possible if the standards of "perfection" are common, reasonable, respected, and agreed upon by both you and your partner. For example, obviously (and not infrequently) you have to provide for the needs of two parties at the same time for the same event. To live happily in a society, it is even worse; you have to deal with so many diverse personalities. This is obvious and self-explanatory.

So, there occasionally comes a time that the ideology about many events in real life may be so different that a compromise is not possible. For instance, two parties may have a dispute about political concepts of capitalism over communism, or on the personal liking of certain sports, music, hobbies, or even the habits of active sexual positioning, etc. But despite the wide range of differences in some aspects of personal life, a communication with a smile, kindness, and an open mind can be so contagious that the gap of difference can be narrowed and diminished; thereby both parties can live with it. If a person's overt attitude of dominance is explosively prevailing, it would be impossible to live together without inflicting some damage to one another. Under this circumstance, they should not live together.

To illustrate this scenario, here is a real story of two urologists who work together, urologist A and B. For some unrevealed reasons, urologist A insists upon performing cystoscopy (a procedure to look into the urinary bladder) on almost all female patients who come to the office, and to do urethral dilation (stretching the urethra or the channel) on every female patients who present themselves with irritative voiding symptoms such as urinary frequency and urgency. Urologist A even repeatedly tells urologist B by saying, "As far as I am concerned, every female patients coming to a urologist's office should have a cystoscopy as long as I do no harm to the patients." However, urologist B will only do cystoscopy for those patients having documented red blood cells in the urine, persistent presence of white blood cells in the urine without documented infection, or refractory bladder irritation without documented urinary tract infection, etc., and almost will never do a urethral dilation on female patients. This is indeed quite a contrast in the concept and practice between these two urologists. However, after they sit down and talk over the innermost secrets of their differences in practice, they are able to respect the concept and practice of one another and continue to work together independently with mutual professional respect and without inflicting harm to the other's dignity and autonomy in medical practice. Of course, urologist A generates more income than urologist B. This is an example of an honorable resolution in real life.

For sexual partners, a similar spirit and practice of mutual understanding and compromise can be exercised. And it is possible, if the standards of being "perfect" are commonly, reasonably and respectfully recognized and honored, and are followed by the same two persons. To explore the understanding, complexity, and fulfillment of the pursuit of perfection as a person, as a couple, or even as a society, let us use the following three examples in life as an "analogy" to illustrate this concept of perfection.

Analogy 1 – A Class Listening to a Melody

Take music as one of the examples of life. Now, let us play a musical tape, or a CD, to a group of one hundred people. Now let us observe what the reactions of each of these one hundred persons may be. Some of these persons, in their own minds, may demand that the music be turned off immediately because they just simply do not like it. Others may be indifferent to listening to the music and do not pay much attention to it. Another group may be really excited with what they hear and they really enjoy the music and even hum along. But, only a very few of the group will really pay complete attention to the music and be able to identify and analyze what instruments are being played and how the melody and the spirit of the music was enacted and personified.

Why do the different groups among these 100 persons have such a wide range of perception of the very same music? Although all of these 100 persons were born with similar instincts and abilities, they still need to go through the process of learning and practicing musical awareness before they can become "good" listeners of music. However, the degree of effort could be widely varied among these 100 people. The result of learning and the abilities that they might have acquired are all quite different as well. And the same is true for many people that try to acquire knowledge about sexuality. The quality and quantity of "effort and ability" will quickly determine one's learning "sensitivity and specificity" of perception and knowledge. What is the difference in the perception of the music among these

100 people? The bottom line is that they have developed different levels of sensitivity and specificity according to their own ability to analyze the music. Even though they may have achieved high levels of sensitivity and specificity in perceiving the music, it will still be forever impossible for them to be "perfect". But a small group from these 100 people will still be at the top level of their sensitivity and specificity in sensing the music. This special group of people will stand out and enjoy most of the music. They are qualified to be called the "artists" of music. And despite their high achievement in music, they may still constantly feel that there is some "shortage" in their life that prevents them from being perfect. Therefore, they will most likely continue to work hard and be eager to improve, maintain, and sustain themselves at the highest levels of sensitivity and specificity. And it is of no doubt that the musician artists would have spent more time and effort in studying and sharpening their ability to perceive the music in their daily chores as compared to most of people. That is why they are clearly better than most people in understanding and appreciating the music. Obviously, dedication in time and effort makes the difference.

Analogy 2 – A Class Drawing Humming Birds
(Another step in the right direction)

After visualizing and understanding the analogy of musicians, let us now look at a scenario of 100 students drawing humming birds. Here we have a group of 100 students in a class for learning how to draw humming birds. They are all given the same materials and the same instruction on how to draw humming birds. Using the same amount of materials and time, and given the same lecture, the students are given an assignment that would be due in one month; they were to draw and submit a personal drawing of humming birds.

Now, after these 100 students are dismissed with their assignment, what would they do out of the class? Will they do the same thing in spite of receiving the same lectures? Of course, no one will be alike in the amount of time they spend in searching and studying the nature, behavior, and lives of humming birds. Also, the degree of effort in practicing and correcting the drawings of humming birds will be quite different. Furthermore, the mood and spirit of sensing and enjoying what they are doing will be so widely various.

Some will do whatever they can to get an access to all the nearby libraries around them to find all the related books they could concerning humming birds and study them more thoroughly. In addition, some students may seek private tutoring to further their study and knowledge of humming birds. Still, others privately continued to learn and practice drawing humming birds through "self-taught" methods. Furthermore, a select few will never be satisfied with what they "could do" and what they have "already accomplished"; for they are the ones that endlessly continue to study and practice their drawing of humming birds with an unrelenting passion to reach the unattainable territory of perfection. The students pursuing perfection are the elite few in the class, they are really at the highest end of the spectrum. They can be honored as the genuine artists of painting or drawing humming birds. And for some others in the class, they may do nothing at all after receiving the same lectures over the same amount of time and going home with the same official assignment. Clearly, this group of students is at the low end of the class in terms of time and effort needed to complete the assignment and submit their drawings of humming birds.

And the rest of the students are those that fall in between both ends of the group in terms of time and effort in their accomplishment in drawing humming birds. Now, a month has passed by and the assignments are due. All 100 students return to class and turn in their assignments. The submitted drawings of humming birds are posted for public viewing. The resulting scores and appreciation of public viewers appear to spread over a very wide range. Some of the drawings are able to vividly reveal the full spirit and likeness of humming birds. A few of the drawings show humming birds as they really are; alive and full of action! These few drawings will easily draw honor and appreciation from the public. And contrary to these very few masterful artists, some of the submitted drawings could not even be recognized as a drawing of birds, not to mention humming birds. And for the remaining students in the class, the result, score, and appreciation of their drawings will fall in between these two extremes.

Ultimately, the goal of a drawing class was to produce a significant amount of "perfect" drawings of humming birds. But the end results were quite different. Why? Because each student had his/her own unique and distinct level of artistic talent and determination. But one thing for sure was that the degree of "personal" dedication in time and effort had been the pivotal point for many of the young artists. The "common factors" that produced a "masterful drawing" was dedication of time, effort, and determination. And in the same sense, a person will become a sensitive, sexual partner if he/she is willing to learn the true methods of sensuality and sexuality through a personal commitment and dedication of time, effort, and determination.

Analogy 3 –Two People Playing a Duet on a Piano

A person's sex life essentially involves a great amount of mental and physical coordination that interacts with another person and/or people; therefore, let us find another example to further illustrate the picture of interaction and coordination, specifically, for a couple in the pursuit and accomplishment of perfect sex.

Now, let us imagine that there are two musicians that agree to play a duet on a piano before a live audience. But prior to their agreement, they must first resolve to master the basic theory of music and to practice the music to be performed; and secondly, they must master all the necessary understanding of the melody that is needed for them to play together.

And, in spite of their high levels of individual achievement in the musical world, they must also get along together through their unique personalities and talents. In doing so, they would have a mutually understandable and acceptable code of communication, especially for their musical performance. They would then need to spend a good amount of time, separately and together, in practicing the assigned melody. Later, in addition to their separate and joint practice, they would have to go through the process of refining their "comfort zone" and "coordination zone" in order to have a brilliant performance on stage!

Now, after such an intense preparation, they had a successful performance and received a standing "bravo" ovation. And as expected, they made the music come alive! The audience accepted and enjoyed the spirit of the music through the duet's smooth coordination of internal communication and external performance.

Often, this type of success is not incidental. Instead, it results from a true and sincere dedication of time, effort, and determination! End results; wonder talent as seen by the masses.

And speaking of talents, the amount of talent needed for drawing, playing an instrument well, or performing sexually, varies from person to person. As to individual talents for any particular activity, they are, of course, quite different, but still require a certain amount of dedication and determination. However, it is a commonly recognized fact that all activities in life are learnable and teachable to a certain degree. Furthermore, the degree of dedication in terms of time and effort will make a tremendous difference in the final achievement and expression of all acquired activities. For a perfect sex life, there is no exception or difference. The full sense and expression of sex life can be as wonderful as those in the arts, as long as the participants are willing to follow the spirit of their talent and pursue the perfection of their art. As expected, through the process of the art of perfection, the final chapter of having "perfect sex" will arrive, at least in its conceptual sense. Through your effort in understanding, practicing, and achieving the essence of "perfect sex" as the artists have achieved in their respective life and job, we should be able to obtain, maintain, and sustain a high level of sensitivity and specificity in communication and coordination for all the activities required for a fulfilling sex life.

Now, are you ready and able to pursue and welcome the materialization of perfect sex? It is not far from you and you can get there as long as you are willing to follow, understand, and read on.

A failure to reach a goal in life often results from a person's ignorance of the basics of success.

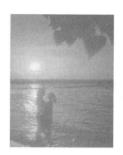

8

Simplified Dynamics of Sexual Performance

Confucius, a Chinese philosopher said, "Food and sex are nature." In part, and in principle, that is correct because we eat to survive and we have sex to reproduce our species from one generation to the next. Today, as we all know, many people are still searching for the ideal answers to their many questions about nutrition and sex. As a result, many different points of view regarding these issues are being reported daily in newspapers and conferences everywhere. Facing a vast host of diversifying opinions, for even the same issue, we sometimes feel that we are getting lost in a maze of varying convictions. Of course, all of these opinions bear much of their own merit and value, but they tend to confuse the "average" person.

At a time when many people are confronting difficulties

in their nutrition and/or sex life or other matters of life, we frequently seek the opinions of experts.

Don't you know that many experts simply come from average people? Much of what is seen and observed is what everyone naturally does in daily life.

For example, even though it is clear that a healthy sex life is a very close part of everyone's daily life, we are often not sure about what we should be enjoying in sex life. Don't you think that such a pattern of taking care of our daily living matters for sex is sometimes petty and inconvenient? Can't we handle, if not all problems, at least most of the problems ourselves that involve sex, instead of heavily relying upon the opinions of experts all the time?

Therefore, let us determine if we can rely upon our "common sense" to help ourselves and only use experts at certain times and during absolutely necessary occasions, not all the time. Please remember to be confident in yourself, after all, we are humans and have common sense! This attitude and approach to sexuality is exactly the way I favor to advise and provide for the caring of my patients with sexual difficulties.

In every phase of sex life, we express what we mean and how we should act in a wide variety of ways. And this may be different from person to person, depending upon their different backgrounds, their family, their education, and all social events in their past experiences. But, in spite of these differences, we all seem to aim at the very same goal; "to fulfill our pursuit of perfection, to satisfy our sexual partners, and to satisfy ourselves." Any success in expressing our sexual behaviors has relied upon our ***mental comfort to perform*** and our ***physical fitness to act***. In order to optimize the combined condition of our mental and physical abilities, we have no choice but to take the responsibility to obtain, maintain, and sustain all the potential factors that will favor our ultimate success in performance. To understand the basic dynamics for performing successfully in any behaviors of life, we must first understand and truly accept the intrinsic dynamics of our "mind and body".

For an easy understanding of this matter, I would like to simplify the intrinsic dynamics for success as follows: Let us consider all the factors that favor our mental comfort to perform collectively as **Factor A**, and those to favor our physical fitness to act as **Factor B**.

For an easy understanding of each factor, let us express them with a number scale from 1 to 10.

Therefore, in order to perform any activities in life well enough to satisfy the standards of persons or society, two minimal requirements must be met: these two minimal requirements can be expressed with the following two formulas:

Formula 1:

Factor A or Factor B should be equal to or more than 4. or Factor A > 4 and Factor B > 4 as well.

Formula 2:

Factor A plus Factor B should be equal to or more than 10. or Factor A + Factor B = > 10.

As you may vividly remember from some of your earlier experiences in life, there were days when you might have felt that you are very smart like "Einstein" and you could do almost anything. And on other days, you simply felt that you were a "dummy" and you just couldn't do anything at all. Ask yourself, "why did I express and behave with such extremes of performance?" And as you would probably agree, it was because you had your good days for many things and you had you bad days for other things in life. But, in reality, all the examples of these two extremes of performance are simply reflecting the end expression of the combined, delicate interaction between your mental comfort to perform and physical fitness to act.

To review the performance of anything you do, let us always go back to the basics and examine what is the combined weight of the mental comfort to perform and the physical fitness to act by using the aforementioned formulas. If you are honest with yourself, you will most likely have no difficulty finding out what went wrong. Let us say one day your mental comfort to perform is less than 4, or say it is only around 3. Under the above definition of significance for Factor A or Factor B, you will not able to do anything right at the level that meets your satisfaction, even though you may be in excellent physical condition. In life, from time to time, the weight of our Factor A and Factor B changes constantly. Usually, for most of people, they are able to manage and handle the weight of Factor A and Factor B within a reasonable limit. Therefore, they can perform well enough to meet the needs of life with various activities. But during the years of a young and productive age, the range of the changing weight of Factor A and Factor B is usually moving within a much wider range as compared to the years of a higher age. In other words, younger people have a wider flexibility for Factor A and Factor B, especially Factor B – physical fitness to act, than do older people.

Now, as you probably remember in your youth, you were

still able to keep going and perform a job well into the next day after an overnight deprivation of sleep. But as age advances, in general, it will naturally take a longer time to recover from a heavy physical drainage. Using a person of fifty years old for example, he/she will probably not be able to perform as swiftly or as smoothly as he/she used to after a sleepless night. This, of course, is a fact of life, which deserves our respect. As you can see, the useful range of Factor A and Factor B is narrowing and their flexibility is shrinking as age increases.

The extensive explanation of the dynamics of the delicate interactions between Factor A and Factor B (as previously discussed) is to stress the importance of respecting Nature and the level of ultimate interaction and the accumulation of mental and physical strengths and abilities. The end result of such an accumulation will affect the overall performance of any activity. As you can sense, any job performance represents an active process of combined mental and physical drainage. And the same is true for sexuality, there is no exception, especially at the phase of sexual intercourse. Now, with your own experience, I am quite sure you will agree that sexual intercourse is a life experience of **"heavy mental and physical drainage"** as well.

Regardless of an individual's intelligence, the mind should be constantly stimulated with personal interests. In order to have something to use and drain, you should maintain a high level of mental and physical reserves to initiate, process, and accomplish the whole course of the sexual acts from beginning to end through indirect foreplay, direct foreplay, sexual intercourse, climax, orgasm, resolution, and recovery.

To apply the effect of this simplified formula to our understanding of sexual performance, let us review the Factor A and Factor B of the following patients:

Patients	Factor A	Factor B	Factor A + B	Result
#1	4	6	10	success
#2	7	2	9	failure
#3	5	6	11	success
#4	4	5	9	failure
#5	8	9	17	success

With the concepts described above, you should have no difficulty in understanding why some men may have a greater degree of difficulty to perform their intimate sexual acts well. Such an understanding will help many men easily walk out of their sexual difficulty. Please read on. I can, and will, help you.

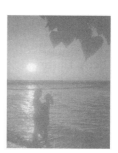

A seamless connection of the parts of a melody will make it unforgettable; so it is for perfect sex.

Phases of a Perfect Sex Cycle

9

The contents of sexuality consist, in fact, of a series of continuous acts, which may be visible or invisible, and verbal or nonverbal. For the purpose of personal and individual understanding, I need to break down these full continuous courses of actions into four phases. They are:

> ***Phase 1:*** ***Indirect foreplay,***
> ***Phase 2:*** ***Direct foreplay,***
> ***Phase 3:*** ***Sexual intercourse, climax and orgasm,***
> ***Phase 4:*** ***Resolution and recovery.***

Phase 1: Indirect Foreplay

The term foreplay has been used to refer to the many variations of mental and physical activities needed before a person attempts a higher, or the very highest, level of sexual intimacy, usually leading to the process of sexual intercourse.

Commonly, one would like to include these activities directly before sexual intercourse. The activities involved can be kissing, caressing, rubbing, pressing, loving and sensual discourse, exciting wording, ...anything that can bring up a feeling of sexual arousal which subsequently leads to the final phase of sexual intimacy through the full course of sexual intercourse. Conceptually, a fulfilling sex life is a matter of continuation, a stream of daily activities with a special orientation towards more sexually explicit acts and expressions, not fragmentation. At its highest moment, men and women will usually experience a series of muscular contractions, especially in the pelvic region, which at the same time come along with the intense feeling of pleasure and subsequent gratification. This brief moment is called *climax*, or an *orgasm*. For men, they will usually have an ejaculation with a series of spurts of semen to complete their orgasm. They then feel a great relief of emotional and physical tension that culminates into total relaxation at the end of sexual intercourse.

In order to progress and reach the moments that begin sexual intercourse, you need to "fine tune" your mental and physical preparation and orientation towards a common goal of eventual sexual intercourse. Your dedication should be much like the audience that listened to the same melody, the artists that drew the humming birds, and the musicians that played a piano duet; there was a "common factor", people working together for a common goal. To be the "best" that they could be, you need common sensitivity and specificity in communication, preparation, and coordination of talent. Therefore, to experience fulfilling and intimate sexual acts, it is imperative that you prepare yourself to be mentally and physically ready for sexual acts. You will then feel you make yourself, as well as your sexual partner, gratified.

And through your repetitive preparations and performances with successful sexual acts, just like those experienced by successful artists, painters or musicians who aim for a more successful performance, you will be experiencing an long-lasting and never-ending improvement of forward progress in the way you think, act, and feel. Sex is an art that you pursue at the highest level of accomplishment. . . and that is the process of perfecting sex and sexuality.

Now, you should be aware of, and have a reasonable understanding of, what "indirect foreplay" is. In general, I refer to it as a phase of building and maintaining a solid interpersonal feeling in the relationship. A deep internal relationship between you and your sexual partner is extremely gratifying when the two of you experience the "whole" course of sexuality, from "indirect" foreplay to the intense sexual intimacy of sexual intercourse.

Also, indirect foreplay begins with your daily activities of living together and caring for each other from moment to moment. This level of interaction is usually limited to verbal, visual, or tactile contacts and interaction with no significant direct physical contacts and exchanges. With your sensorial alertness and a high sensitivity and specificity of all your senses, you will be able to conduct effective communication with your sexual partner. In time, the affection between you and your sexual partner will develop into an attraction from which you will be emotionally and physically rewarded. Further advancement towards a closer relationship is the next natural and progressive step of a special expression of appreciation. And within such a course of effort and interaction, you will have developed an interpersonal relationship. And this, in itself, will prepare you for the next phase of mastering perfect sex; "direct foreplay".

For a couple that successfully experiences indirect foreplay, usually they will have a strong feeling that they cannot wait for the upcoming right time, right place, and right situation to open up before their "direct foreplay" commences.

Phase 2: Direct Foreplay

Direct foreplay is a group of more explicit mental and physical actions. Known as "foreplay of sexual intercourse", they are usually described and noted in many circulating books or contemporary magazines. Direct foreplay may consist of all the varieties of direct physical contacts in addition to mental comfort. The actions involved may be soft kissing, slow caressing, gentle rubbing against each other, sensually touching and stimulating, and any means that you are able to create and imagine, as long as the concerns of your sexual partner's mental and physical well being is kindly considered, respected, practiced, and protected. In other words, you can act whatever way you can imagine but you will want to come to a mutual agreement. From there, the fire of compassion and sexual excitement is igniting, developing, and spreading. Furthermore, both of you will eagerly demand more and more sexual excitement to feel and appreciate one another and to eventually proceed further at a higher level of intimacy with sexual intercourse.

This is the magic of effective and sensible direct foreplay. Again, you did a good job on this part of sexuality. Now, are you ready to go all the way to a world that will allow you to enjoy the highest level of sexual intimacy?

Phase 3: Sexual Intercourse, Orgasm, and Ejaculation

As sexual emotion and excitement evolve, develop, and advance through the magical power of the actions taken place in Phase 1 and Phase 2, you will naturally reach an uncontrollable urge and desire for sexual intercourse in conjunction to the action and harmony of the feeling. Every act of sexual intercourse requires a simultaneous full devotion and concentration from you and your sexual partner in order to capture and enjoy the full body and spirit of physical sensation and mental gratification. Such a delicate action and feeling only comes from continuous vaginal penetration that culminates, usually, within two to five minutes with a series of muscular contractions, especially in the pelvic region and with a stream of intense pleasure. This is an orgasm. Men will have an ejaculation of semen, the penile erection will subside, and the entire body relaxes into a peaceful state of "perfect sexual appeasement".

Therefore, the sooner you can imagine yourself and your sexual partner starting on this journey, the sooner you will fulfill all of your delicate and intimate phases of "sexual life cycles" over and over. Through repetitive gratification and rewarding sexual experiences with your sexual partner, the depth of your sexual coordination and concentration will be naturally intensified and sustained.

Phase 4: Resolution and Recovery

After your sexual partner and you have reached mutual orgasm with the feeling of the highest level of pleasure and gratification, it is imperative that you and your sexual partner share a period of time to relax, hug, and gently caress and converse. And both of you can enjoy sensing the wonder of mutual appreciation and commitment to life.

And sooner than you could imagine, another cycle of a sexual journey will begin to further enhance the quality and quantity of life of your sexual partner and you. With such a fine detailed action and operation of sex life as we just shared together, I have no doubt that your life will be greatly enriched.

Although the phases of sexual cycles are identified and subdivided into the four phases as described above, it would be beneficial for you to think of the "whole picture" of perfect sex as a course of visible, invisible, verbal, and nonverbal acts with a smooth continuous transition between each phase. It is more like a beautiful picture of the playing of wonderfully orchestrated music in which the transition of various sections of the melody can be identified, and the coordination of the playing of all instruments may be enjoyably verified and appreciated.

To acquire the wisdom and instinct for "perfect sex", it takes the willingness of the participants to obtain, maintain, and sustain an awareness of the unique forms and phases of communication. Furthermore, one must become sensitive to all forms of language: body language, verbal and nonverbal, mood swings, facial expressions, physical and nonphysical communication, etc. Thereby, you and your sexual partner will be able to follow every phase through a series of mutually agreeable and coordinating actions, journeying towards the goal of "perfect sex" from beginning to end.

Now we are making a great advancement towards our intended "perfect sex" by enriching the quality of life, by observing life's subtle signals, and by becoming acutely aware of life's daily living.

A common value to respect and follow is the key for people to work together.

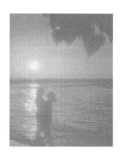

10

Principles to Reach Perfect Sex

As we previously described, the mental and physical actions and interactions of a good sex life are the matters of the individual and/or the couple, but its eventual value is very far-reaching for all people in all societies. Sex is a non-verbal and invisible gluing power of couples and societies. It is the single most contributing factor for harmony in the life of individuals, couples, and societies as well. Therefore, while individual enjoyment and freedom in life is increasingly, and intensely, entertained in our society, the effect of sex life upon life, communities, individuals, and entire populations cannot be denied or ignored. Right or wrong, sex has infiltrated every form of public media: television, movies, radio, music, magazines, newspapers, textbooks, billboards, etc. Consequently, the interpretation of its message is left to the "viewer". I cannot deny or ignore my obligation as a doctor to reassure, explain, and counsel my patients and readers that sex is not dirty or evil, but it is the fulfillment of life! Please be aware that the following information is about "perfecting" sexuality and what I have shared with my patients and their family members through my private medical practice. Their endorsement and improvement in personal sex life is direct proof that my intent and practice has, and will, benefit you to perfect your own sex life in a sensible, safe, and responsible way.

And the perfection of your sex life can be reached under the concepts that I have previously described. To discuss the principle to perfecting sex life, we must thoroughly think about, and consider, the following questions, and practice the essence of the reasonable answers and outcomes to these questions. Therefore, the questions are as follows (and please answer them honestly in your own mind):

1. *With "whom" are you going to enjoy, or want to express, your sex life?*

2. *Is there a "special time" when you will reveal your sexual intentions?*

3. *Have you chosen a "special place" where you desire to express your sexual intimacy?*

4. *Do you bring a "mutual respect" for your sexual partner? And how will you "express" or signify your sexual intent?*

5. *If necessary, have you taken strict precautions against contracting or spreading sexually transmitted diseases for your sexual partners and yourself?*

The answers to these questions shall be the same. Theoretically, as fully "free" individuals of individualism, you can do whatever you want to do according to your will. However, if what you believe is different from the "proven norm" and the recognition towards ethical relationships with your family members, friends, colleagues, and all other members of your race, society, and country, then please be aware that your decision will strongly effect and guide you to what you should do responsibly. And in answering these questions, it is always important and sensible to bear in mind that the consequences of what you do and what you experience in your sex life will eventually enhance and/or destroy the quality and quantity of your personal, family, and social life.

If what you do fails to generate significant weight or influence for you and your sexual partner to reach a suitable goal, certainly it would not be advisable for you to proceed with such a sexual relationship. If you are not sure, your reluctant sexual acts will eventually be proven in time to be disturbing and even self-destroying for the life of your sexual partner and yourself. Therefore, many of my views represent the majority of people in the main stream of society.

My views do not represent some fragmentation of a "weird fantasy", "fixation", and /or "sexual obsession" that has been practiced among certain groups of people in every society. These "special groups" of people are generally tolerated, but not emulated in a normal society.

1. With "whom" are you going to enjoy or want to express your sex life?

That will depend on how liberal you are as to the ethical standards in assessing the value of a relationship with anyone around you. In general, you should not want to have intimate sexual acts with your parents, siblings, and/or direct relatives. Traditionally, it seems a common respected fact among most societies that you would not practice an intimate sexual relationship with any members of your own family. And genetically, it is not advised to do so because it is a fact that there is a higher possibility of developing hereditary diseases.

However, within the truth of real life, sometimes during certain stages of the development of sexuality, someone in the family may have some sexual fantasy toward another family member. But they should be able to control and discipline themselves without any sort of verbal or physical aggressive act that expresses their sexual desire. This phenomenon between parent and child is known as the *Oedipus Complex*. In real life, it is considered to be a normal and an understandable growing process during a certain period of a person's life. At times, a conflicting mental state between the values of respect, morals, and ethics, and sexual feelings and admirations may surface and appear as so-called "Oedipal conflicts". But usually, through the child's conscious and subconscious learning and the awareness of these values, the mind's inherent reasoning values will resolve the "Oedipus complex" without any noticeable effect. If it does become evident, there is no reason to fear one's responses or to be jealous of the child. The child should be shown gently, but firmly, that the physical intimacy of parents is reserved for one another. Meanwhile, the child's attitude towards sexuality should be accepted, and the parents should help the child defer and eventually direct sexual interest toward a different partner or some other outlet.

Sexual relationships among family members is known as *incest*, which is a very complicated issue among most races and societies. The discussion of further details is beyond the limit and scope of the "original purpose" in writing this book.

As a practicing urologist, who has dedicated his time and effort in helping many men and women with their sexual difficulties on a day to day basis, to continue the discussion of incest would simply detract from my "intent and purpose" for writing this book. Simply be aware that sexual intimacies among blood relatives should not be accepted, or tolerated, as normal behavior.

Who is the "RIGHT" person for you to engage in an intimate sexual relationship? Based on the above discussion, I do not believe that you will find any difficulties in making a fine and final decision for the benefit of family, society, and yourself. Who is "RIGHT" for you? The essence of "truth" to this question lies within the "personal taste" of each individual. Each person should evaluate interests, likes/dislikes, emotional and physical stimulation, dedication and determination of goals, the sense and expression of sexuality, satisfaction, mental and physical coordination of mind and spirit, and then simply use "common sense". In other words, allow "wisdom" to be your counterpart in decision-making.

2. Is there a "special time" when you will reveal your sexual intentions?

To most people, it is easy to allow their common sense to tell them when they may perform sexual acts in different situations, places, and/or times such as vacations, hotels, motels, secret rendezvous, etc. However, sometimes you may find a small minority of people who are obsessed with a "fantasy place" for some unusual public exposure of their sexual acts, and this could lead to problems.

In general, any form of a sexual act could, and should, carry its far-reaching and beneficial effect to enrich the quality and quantity of one's personal life, family life, and/or social life. But to the contrary, any sexual act that may cause a disturbance and an embarrassment to anyone around you should be severely discouraged. Although you may say that you have your rights, your full freedom to do whatever you want to do under the Constitution of the United States of America, there is still a fine line of reality that exists between "can do it" and "should not do it" which you need to observe and respect. Therefore, it is clear, and important, for you to express your sexual acts to conform within the levels of relationships of your surroundings.

After all, it is your solemn responsibility to express your sexual desires and acts at the right time and at the right degree. In public, you feel comfortable with gently kissing one another. You probably would not feel appropriate and comfortable having sexual intercourse in public or in front of your family. However, there are some people that claim deviant sex thoughts and/or actions are sexually stimulating and exciting.

On a personal level, each individual seems to have their own "right time" or "best time" to sense their sexual desires and express their sexual acts. For example, someone may like to have sexual intercourse before falling asleep and someone else may prefer to have a sexual intercourse after a good night's sleep. While a personal preference in selecting a time-frame for sexual act does exist, it is more reasonable and advisable for a couple to find a common ground of a mutually preferred time in terms of their preparation of mental and physical conditions. In doing so, a mutual comfort zone can be secured and there will be no feelings of disappointment from being reluctant in choosing the right or wrong time to have explicit sexual acts in the privacy of their own time.

3. *Have you chosen a "special place" where you desire to express sexual intimacy?*

Obviously, the choice of a right place to enjoy sex life is equally as important as compared to the right time and with the right person. The variation of choices for a place to enjoy sex can be unlimited because there are so many variables in the degree of sexual acts. As you can sense, and imagine, there are even more variations when we combine the consideration of time, person, and place together to make a final choice clearly because they all interact in some sense with one another. However, the bottom-line decision is to ask yourself; "If what I do, and how I do it, does not hurt or harm anyone, but will enhance the quality of my life and sexual partner's life, how can this be wrong?" As a doctor, I am not here preaching to you. Instead, I am just reminding you of common sense for personal and social responsibility. Although, at times, you have read about or seen at the movies or even on television "talk shows" that depict highly graphic sexual acts in front of people as someone's fantasy and excitement, this is, after all, the exception for the majority of people in the main stream of society. There is an enormous difference between "thinking about it" and "acting about it". Sexual deviations do exist among some people; they are not the "norm" of society.

The goal of an individual's sexuality has been well defined throughout this discussion. In short, a satisfactory sex life will enhance the quality of an individual's life through repetitive, successful experiences in the performance of sexual acts at all phases (indirect foreplay, direct foreplay, sexual intercourse, orgasm, resolution and recovery) as previously described. If each experience in your sex life is repeated with the same "perfect satisfaction", I am then quite sure that you will begin to understand my premise of "Perfect Sex"!

Please remember that while you are making love "with your sexual partner", you must remain honest with yourself. You must generate the "ultimate mental and physical pleasure" for your sexual partner's needs, and not just for yourself; this is the basic "number one" concept towards satisfying a sexual partner.

4. How will you "express" or signify your sexual intents? How are you going to act and enjoy a sex life with your sexual partner?

To answer this compound question, I would suggest that you and your sexual partner become equally aware of your mutual feelings; it involves the attitude of "to give" and "to be given" or "to receive." Both partners must learn to share emotions, desires, wants, and needs. In other words, both must learn to openly and effectively communicate by any forms, or means, that are comfortable for them. And you can attain and develop this skill of communication easily.

With the skills of effective communication in hand, you still need to give someone, presumably being the right person, what you have and do so in the ways that she/he would want to enjoy at the right time, right place, and right manner. That is "to give" something to someone in the way she/he wants to be given, not just to give her/him what you have. If this practice is not properly undertaken, the outcome and ultimate effects of your sexual acts will not be long lasting, never-ending, or fruitful as they are intended to be.

To accomplish this, we need to go back to the original

basic principle for sound and proper communication at a high level of sensitivity and specificity, which is constantly required in any of the levels and stages of a gratifying sex life.

5. Safe Sex: If necessary, have you taken strict precautions against contracting or spreading sexually transmitted diseases to your sexual partner(s) as well as yourself ?

Any disease has the potential to impose a substantial adverse effect on someone's mental and physical aspects of life. And as we know, many diseases can be transmitted through intimate sexual acts. The ultimate and damaging effects may range from significant mental anguish to even death.

The examples of sexually transmitted diseases are:

1. **By virus**
   - Genital herpes infection
   - Genital warts (condyloma acuminata)
   - Molluscum contagiosum
   - Hepatitis
   - AIDS

2. **By bacteria**
   - Gonorrhea
   - Syphilis
   - Nongonococcal urethritis (NGU)
   - Chancroid
   - Lymphogranuloma venereum, also known as tropical bubo
   - Granuloma inquinale
   - Vaginal infection

3. By protozoa
   • Trichomonas –"trich"

4. By parasite – lice or mites
   • Pediculosis pubis (by crab lice)
   • Scabies (by a mite)

5. By fungus
   • Candidiasis – also known as thrush or monilia

Of course, the details of all these diseases are beyond the scope and sequence as intended for the original goal of this book. The purpose of listing them is not to show you how much a doctor knows, but to make you aware of the fact that there are a wide variety of diseases caused by sexual contacts. The ones that are more commonly seen in my practice are nongonococcal urethritis, genital warts, genital herpes, and gonorrheal urethritis. They can be treated effectively, most of time, without many severe residual effects. But some diseases, such as AIDS and hepatitis can be severe enough to cause death.

The key point in treatment is to be sure that sexual partners are treated at the same time with close attention and a follow-up exam by your doctor. Failure to do so is a common reason for recurrence. Therefore, please be sure to be cooperative with your doctor's advice. But be careful not let an occasional dishonest medical professional take advantage of your anxiety and fear and submit you to a lot of tests; especially those that are done in their office.

For the purpose of perfecting your sex life, I would like to share with you a story that has a common scenario:

Some years ago, a gentleman came to see me with a great amount of anxiety and fear. He was very concerned about a pus discharge from his urine opening (urethral meatus). Apparently, he had spent several days in Las Vegas, and while he was there, he had visited a house of prostitution. Upon his returning home, he suddenly discovered an infection, accompanied with a pus discharge from his channel. I then treated him successfully with appropriate antibiotics after a few basic studies. Fortunately, his wife was willing to have the same treatment at the same time. This couple had no long-term ill effect from the infection. This gentleman was very frightened of this disease and was extremely worried about the possibility of giving this disease to his wife. He did not know how to explain the situation to his wife. Subsequently, he confessed that he had a fight with his wife, he got mad and left for Las Vegas. I told him that this is the price that you are sometimes responsible to pay. I asked him to be honest and brave and that he must speak to his wife about this most serious problem. In this case, he did, and both received treatment timely, both were cured, and I was very happy that they did so well.

Here, I would like sincerely to caution anyone who is interested in, or may have already indulged in, intimate sexual acts with prostitutes or multiple sexual partners. Please be aware of the following facts. Most certainly, it is highly probable that a stranger who is willing to perform intimate sexual acts (intercourse) with you will easily do the same with others as well. The more sexual partners a person has, the greater the risk becomes for contracting a sexually transmitted disease. And for treatment and follow-up, the exposure to multiple sexual partners by more than two parties will definitely make simultaneous treatments for all the sexual partners extremely difficult. Understandably, it is easier to treat and track down one couple than it is to track down multiple sexual partners in an endless cycle of sex games.

Therefore, although multiple sexual encounters seem quite entertaining and interesting to imagine, it is no fun to contract sexually transmitted diseases with even more difficult conditions to eliminate and control. In addition, such a practice can generate a great deal of mental and physical stresses for all sexual partners involved. All of these unfavorable effects are endless; and you are the only one that can decide what you should do, and practice, in your own personal sex life.

For perfecting your own sex life, this basic understanding of the consequence suffered from contracting and spreading sexually transmitted diseases should not be lightly overlooked. How to accomplish and materialize your dream of perfecting sex life is within your reach by following the details previously discussed. I wish you luck and success in your pursuit of a perfect sex life.

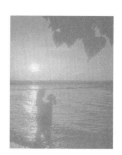

An example with fact and unique prominence is unforgettable for learning.

11

A Contemporary Case Study

After we have learned the **criteria for "perfect sex"**, that is, to have a sexual relationship with the right person at a right time and in a right place, with the right manners, mutual respect, and safety, now is the time to find an example for illustration. Due to the enormous publicity of President Clinton's sex affairs, my searching mind naturally came to the story of his sex scandals. In addition, in our American history there has never been a similar sex scandal involving a politician that has been scrutinized so intensely with a sense of politics, ethics, and morality and received such a notoriety of publicity.

While the real sense of being right or wrong is a personal matter, the common sense that prevails in an existing society can help people forge a direction of general sentiment and righteousness. Up to this moment, the "real truth" of the details of President Clinton's personal sexual affairs might still be far from its full revelation. However, the general public has learned thus far a vast amount of information from various media such as newspapers, magazines, TV, the Internet, or radio shows, including President Clinton's personal confession. Based on the available information from various angles, what is your score card for President Clinton's performance of "perfect sex"? Of course, it is up to your discretion. However, we should not ignore his political job achievements as our President.

Hence, as a common part of our daily national conversation, it has become inevitable for people to talk about our President's sex affair. On a comfortable summer morning in 1998, there were six male professionals sitting in a lounge and talking about President Clinton's sex scandal (which has been viewed as a soap opera in America and in the world).

One of the six, sitting in a couch, sighed and said, "How come President Clinton is so horny?"

The one in front of the first speaker quickly replied, "What is wrong with being horny? We men are all horny anyway, aren't we? You, too."

The one on the right side inserted and said, "Wait a minute! What did you say? I don't get horny."

However, the one sitting at the left-end corner of the lounge with his legs crossed, spoke out slowly with the wisdom of an experienced senior, "Every man has testosterone to help develop his manhood. It is no exception for President Clinton, and he has a lot of male hormone as any other man does. Being horny is not all that bad. As a matter of fact, it is a blessing from God for the man as well as for his sexual partner, as long as he behaves and interacts with a right person in a right way at a right time and place, and also with mutual respect and safety. But we still don't really know if everything reported was true and how he did it."

His talk stirred a serious look from others and induced a wave of laughter. At the end, almost everyone nodded and said, "That's right."

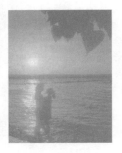

An effective discipline and habit will do wonders for life. The detailed scenes of the actions by any successful humans in life are the good examples; no exception.

12
Secrets of Obtaining a Perfect Sex Life

From your efforts of going through the above sections, you should have a good comprehension of what you can, and should, do to perfect your sex life. After that, it is a matter of dedication and practice, from which the effects of reconditioning and forming new habits will emerge for your daily use. And it is all up to you. The following steps are what I would recommend for anyone who wants to follow a perfect sex life:

1. Communication with High Sensitivity and Specificity

The secret of obtaining a perfect sex life begins with the ability to have sensitive, open, and specific lines of communication between individuals. No two individuals are alike. But in spite of the existence of individual difference in talents, personalities, likes, and dislikes, the true formula of "success" remains the same because the path of human behaviors, in essence, remains constant as well.

The basic and essential truth for successful and meaningful communication begins when the speaker's "wants and needs" are clearly and specifically stated. In this way, an individual receiving the information will naturally have a greater chance to understand the clarity of the message. A successful and/or dysfunctional communication between two individuals is, within a reasonable limit, quite constantly traceable.

On numerous occasions in my practice of sex counseling, many patients and/or their partners have related the following complaints to me by saying, "I don't know why, but before we were married, I simply blinked my eyes or waved my hands, he/she knew exactly what I meant right away... Now, after all these years of living together, he/she doesn't seem to know what I'm talking about.... I can yell in his/her ears, and he/she still doesn't know what I mean.... I get so angry!"

Does this scenario in life sound all too familiar to you? This is a real life situation for many couples. And it clearly illustrates a deterioration of communication skills that cause a gradual loss of sensitivity and specificity during their discussions of sexual "wants and needs." Unfortunately, for some couples, there is a breakdown in communication skills after a few years of living together. They have taken communication for granted. They did not keep up their high alertness to listen to, and to understand, one another as they did before living together. Therefore, in order to reestablish an effective communication channel between a couple, this basic, essential requirement of open, effective communication should be reinforced into their daily actions of living together. In failing to do so, there is no hope to improve the quality of "indirect foreplay", which is the basic foundation for further involvement, improvement, and advance in one's sex life. Without effective communication, which is intended as indirect foreplay, further actions in sexual relationships tends to take place under unfair conditions with some reluctance from either party, or tends to be "one-sided". This situation will make intercourse, in a strict sense, be suspected as a forced act, or just like a rape. Although a momentary sexual pleasure may be experienced through instinctive responses, this will not benefit the quality of one's future life and/or sexual relationship. Instead, it will make the relationship and quality of life deteriorate.

Therefore, maintaining and sustaining a high awareness of sensitivity and specificity is the first step, and the absolute requirement, that is needed to restore the lost and effective communication skills that an active, sexual couple once found so natural and easy. It is that simple of a secret! Clear and precise communication will not be misunderstood or misconstrued. Sexual "wants and needs" will not be interpreted incorrectly. Thus, sexual partners will be on the correct path, moving towards their goal, a goal of "perfect sex".

2. Imagination and Exploration

When a couple makes a decision to get married, or a decision to live together for a long period of time, no matter what the decision is, a couple will eventually, and inevitably, be faced with the many realities of daily life. When the problems and questions begin, does this mean that this is the end of the highest momentum of a relationship, a relationship that they had built before they decided to live together or to get married? I hope not, but it is true that the realities and routines of daily life will consume much of a person's time and energy. This may also make some couples overlook their need for continuing their efforts to maintain and sustain the delicacy of their interpersonal relationship as they did before getting together. Instead, it would be more beneficial for them to imagine that living together, married or unmarried, is just the beginning of really falling in love. If the spirit and feeling of falling in love are to automatically prevail in one's daily living, a higher level of sensitivity and specificity in communication during every stage of one's sex life should be naturally nurtured, maintained, and sustained. You may riddle me and say that I'm too idealistic or naive, but do you have a better way?

At one time during my practice, I saw an eighty-six year old man, a farmer. He came to me because of a problem he had with slow urine flow. As I took his medical history, he also mentioned that he has slowed down quite a bit in his sexual responses over the past five years. I inquired about who has been his sexual partner and he said it is his wife. I further asked him how the quality of their sex life and marriage has been. This inquiry made him smile and reply, "Our sex life and marriage have been perfect. We love it."

Whenever a couple tells me of their "great affection" for each other, I always asks my patients, "What is your secret?" The eighty-six year old farmer was no exception, so I asked him, "What is your secret formula for a perfect sex life and marriage?" He said with a smile, "I would say 'Honey, I love you,' and then I hug her, or embrace her, or simply touch her at least three times every day before we go to bed at the end of a day. We keep ourselves healthy this way...." As he was leaving my office, I noticed that his wife was sitting in the waiting room of my office. I congratulated them for their great achievement in life. She smiled and confirmed her husband's confession. "Quite an impressive story!" I thought to myself. It could be a role model for anyone who wishes to have a good marriage with a good sex life as well. What this couple has been doing for their sixty-five years of marriage is still as romantic as what they did before they got married.

Therefore, it is advisable to imagine that the moment a couple decides to live together is simply the beginning of another story of falling in love. In such a sense, it would be thought that the task of sustaining a good relationship with a sexual partner is one of the priorities of life. Naturally, one should be willing to spare enough time and energy for your partner to do as many things as possible together. With such a constant intent and practice, it is sure that the couple will appreciate one another on a daily basis. As to how a couple should share the feelings and how they should sustain their high intensity of mutual attention, I can only suggest that it is within the imagination, trust, and exploration of both people as long as you both agree, and believe, that there is no limitation to romance and understanding.

Technically, you have all the tools such as the senses and abilities of hearing, smelling, touching, seeing, and imagining for you to use. To a natural sense, whatever you do that can enhance the quality of a relationship should be worthwhile for you to explore further, and to keep. The pattern and variation of your using all these tools are clearly, and freely, at your disposal. If you discover a sense of rhythm that can serve both you and your sexual partner well, you have my congratulations. Preserve and enrich it, for perfection is like a lullaby for a baby.

3. Repetition

While you discover and capture a rhythm, or a formula, that can well serve you and your sexual partner, you are wise to take a step further to refine it. From that time on, repetition is the key to success. Having a wonderful sex life, being a sensitive person, developing effective communication skills, and striving for perfection, all of these things closely resemble the scenario of a musician on stage playing for an audience. The musician knows that he/she can never stop practicing because repetition makes perfection; but it also makes the pursuit easier and more enjoyable to perform.

In the previously stated story about the eighty-six year old farmer, it should be noted that the farmer and his wife repeated the same main course with success to express their affections toward one another for over sixty-five years. Did he feel bored? Apparently not. Otherwise, how could they have enjoyed living together and being sexual partners for over sixty-five years?

4. Perfection

Repetition with intention and action to perfect one's self-awareness is the same attribute and passion that many artists have cultivated throughout the ages.

In music, design, literature, etc., it is the heart and spirit of the artists to explore, experience, and perfect their artworks. For one's sex life, you will soon become an **artist of your own sex life** if you apply the same endeavor that artists do for their works.

To sum up, I would like to share some "secrets" of many responsible, fulfilling couples have possessed and commonly told me for their marriage and sex life as follows:

"I have to listen to what she/he says...." or

"Sometimes, I like to play dumb...." or

"We both really enjoyed our sex life...." or

"We never let our anger go to bed with us...." or...

"My husband never uses a rough word or act to me...." or

"He is always kind, gentle in his words and acts for me...." or

"We are always able to find something to do together...."
or

"She is a lovely lady. She always likes to touch and look at me...." or

"I like to touch my wife a few times before going to bed...."
or

"I like to be a good student of 'Honey-Do' College...."

I hope that these sampled statements should be easy for you to capture the essence of the spirit and practice of perfect sex and life. At the end, there is no real secret for perfect sex. In fact, the fulfillment of one's "perfect" sex and life merely results from a combined use of common sense, sensitive and specific communication, commitment, devotion, sacrifice, kindness, smiles, gentle acts, repetition, and perfecting your identified formula. And perfect sex is yours to grasp, use, and enjoy forever.

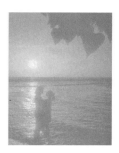

Perfecting is the absolute attribute of artists and only it can steer them to the wonderland of perfection.

13

Artistic View of Sex Life

Mentally, a person always has many gaps that exist between the many aspects of the mind and the environment that she/he lives in. The environment can just be anywhere in the world. The gaps urge a person to fill them up; otherwise, she/he will not be in harmony with the environment and will feel restless for another change.

To reach a momentary balance of a person's mental state, our bodies are going through constant changes in order to adjust in many visible and invisible ways. Thereby, you live in a reasonable, comfortable state of balance. If there is a failure to do so, the body will feel uneasy and will need to make a change again. The degree, speed, and skill of making a change may vary from moment to moment and from person to person. That is why every person behaves differently. However, no matter what the difference is, the ultimate goal of making such changes is to reach a balanced and harmonious state of the mind.

The ability to change in order to reach perfection is the accumulation of all that has been learned in the life of a person. In general, the more sensitive and specific the ability of observation, understanding, and communication, the more a person will learn. The more capable a person is to make a smooth, swift, and effective change, the easier it is for the person to adjust and fill the gaps around him. And ultimately, the person's life will be much in harmony and peace with the environment. This process of living is naturally understandable for reaching the wonderland of perfection.

In life, a person cannot do anything about whatever happened in the past. However, the process of learning should never end. It would never be too late to learn and change. Of course, a person will be willing to make a change only when she/he is able to perceive the value of change.

Successful artists are always sensitive and specific in their observations and will show the results of their observations by the corresponding change in their thoughts and acts. They exercise and explore their imagination to create a sense of their own world of harmony and perfection and to display their state of mind in paintings, music, sculptures, etc. The scale and value of their artistic works is judged and revealed by the amount of the appreciation from the existing society. Whether they are appreciated or not, they graciously accept the response from the public and digest their feeling of satisfaction, or frustration, for the future betterment of their works.

However, there is a different point that is worthwhile for us to note; sometimes the art works of an artist could not be well recognized and appreciated during his/her lifetime because his/her vision was far beyond the reach of the contemporary public. But this artist might have the ability, and the courage, to endure the ignorance of the environment. And his/her art works can go unnoticed until it is recognized years or generations later. However, the artistic work of a man's sex life can not go unnoticed without an adverse effect, or feedback. Instead, it demands an instant reward and appreciation.

To explore and create your own contents of a perfect sex life, it is most advisable to trust your natural instincts to guide you to the initial and effective step of perfecting your sex life. As you know, most people have all the five basic senses of hearing, seeing, touching, tasting, and smelling. Trust what these senses tell you and simply react to them accordingly, ***but follow the principle that the enjoyment of sex life is to enhance the quality of life for both partners and should not be completed at the expense of someone's pain and suffering.*** By applying the skills of an artist in observing and acting for their creation of art, you too can succeed in creating your own art works of perfect sex.

Here is my congratulation to you for having made an effort to possess the idea and spirit for perfect sex. Now is the time to imagine yourself as an artist, to be on stage to perfect your sex life as musicians on stage do for their audiences. The relation of the contents, spirit and practice between your sex life and the art works of musicians are clearly illustrated in Part III, Section 10 (page 59). And the performance on stage for musicians, and sexual intercourse for men, have been commonly recognized as the final, and peaking, moment to show off their abilities.

Musicians dedicate time and effort to learn and master

their art works, and have spirit, knowledge, and skills to act with the instruments at their disposal. For perfecting a man's sex life, the process of preparation for spirit, skill, and performance for his art works in sex life is not different from a musician for music.

After a man has gone through the stage of preparation with the art of indirect foreplay, now he is ready to act with all the "instruments" at his disposal. You may ask, "What are my instruments for my art works of sex life?" Please imagine that all your sensing abilities, including hearing, seeing, smelling, tasting and touching, as well as all your moving abilities, are all your available instruments at your disposal. In other words, every sense and act could be the available instrument that you can apply for the benefits of you and your sexual partner. Furthermore, imagine that you are on a mission for your audience, that is, your sexual partner is a special person to perceive your art works. The final output and performance to please you and your sexual partner is just like the wonderful music for the frenzied audience from a successful, yet sensitive, musician.

Now you understand the spirit and practice of artistry. As well, you know what and where your instruments are for expressing sexual feelings and acts. The next step for you is to learn how to use them at the right time, in a right way, and in a right combination. While a certain melody could be very pleasing and you would like to listen to it over and over, it is a great idea however to once in a while be creative in composing and performing your sexual melody with all the resources as previously described. In doing so, the width and depth of your sex life will be ever expanding without tiredness. As a result, you will have a more fulfilling product of sex life for you and your sexual partner to appreciate.

Part IV

●

Sexual Difficulties in Men

"A result from the failure and frustration in sex life has ruined many men's life. Yet today's concept, skill, and technique in managing sexual difficulty in men have brought the light of its resolution. A man's happy time can continue to be compatible with his mind and body. Don't worry."

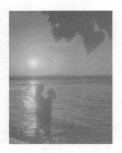

If there is a magical way to get a
job done well, it is a sure readiness
of the basic ingredients for that job;
no shortcut.

14
Basic Requirements for
Good Sexual Performance?

The performance of an intimate sexual act is basically
not different from the requirements needed to perform well
on a job, in a sport, or any other activity in life. As you
know, doing anything in life is a process of mental and/or
physical drainage, which will recover in time. For sexual
intercourse, the same scenario prevails. Fortunately, after
the completion of the wonderful act – sexual intercourse,
men are able to regain their needed mental and physical
resources in time for future repeated use.

Briefly speaking, in order to perform well in intimate
sexual acts, a satisfactory readiness of mental comfort to
perform and physical fitness to act is essential and mandatory.
The details of the basic requirements for a good sex performance were presented in the Section 8, *Simplified Dynamics*

of Sexual Performance in Part III, **The Road to Perfect Sex**. In general, if anything goes wrong, it would be most useful to go back and examine the basics for the failed task before you stick your head into a swamp of confusion and anxiety. Many times, what you might discover is simply that you have missed the basics for completing the task. Therefore, this section just serves as a reminder for anyone who experienced frustration in his sexual performance.

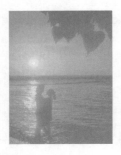

*K*nowing and admitting "what is the difficulty?" is the beginning of correction and improvement.

15
What are the
Sexual Difficulties in Men?

Now, let us look into the causes for men's sexual difficulties. But let us start out with a discussion on the proposed definitions and the terms related with male sexual difficulties, which you might have confronted in many of your prior readings on the related subjects.

Difficulty is a word that we use to describe the frustration resulting from failing to achieve our intended goals of doing something in life. To define the difficulty for an event, we would need to clearly know what are the intended goals of that event. For the same token, I would use ***sexual difficulties in men*** **to describe the frustration that men would experience from failing to achieve their common goals of sex life — generating mutual satisfaction and enhancing quality of life** as we previously defined.

In our contemporary sense of human sexuality, as previously discussed and concluded in Parts I and III, I assume that we all agree on the goals of sexuality being to enhance the quality of the lives of both sexual partners, and is not just for the primitive value of procreation. If men fail to accomplish and materialize this commonly recognized goal, they are simply not doing their job right. And these men have some forms of *sexual difficulty*, involving either mental comfort to perform, or physical fitness to act, or both in combination.

However, you may have been confused by the use of various terms to describe men's concern over their poor sexual performance while you have read the related subjects on sex. For example, *male impotence, erectile disturbance, and erectile dysfunction (ED), sexual problems, sexual dysfunction* and *sexual difficulties* have all been used. The term of **male impotence** tends to deliver a sense of humiliation by berating men's sexual ability; it is emotional and traumatic. However, its frequent use has dulled such a feeling but is still frequently encountered. The terms, *erectile disturbance* and *erectile dysfunction*, virtually, describe the same concern of men over their impaired ability to initiate, maintain, or sustain an erection to complete a sexual intercourse. However, both carry, and reveal, a stronger technical and functional aspect of the erection of the penis for the importance of human sexuality. Recently, *erectile dysfunction* (ED) is more explicitly recommended for medical literature and considered as being more technically to the point.

How about these three terms, *sexual problems, sexual dysfunctions,* or *sexual difficulties?* Although *erectile dysfunction* is used to specifically describe the concern over any problem with penile erection, these three terms all imply a wider range of the problems that men may experience in their sexual performance and that usually result in some anxiety and frustration. However, the term, *sexual difficulties in men*, is less technical, more general, more descriptive, and more familial to most people, especially laypersons. To ease the confusion over the use of so many terms in discussing sexual issues, I choose to use *sexual difficulties* to generally cover the problems of men's sexual practice and *erectile difficulties* to specifically cover men's concern over their no, or poor, erection. Why? It is because the word, *difficulty* carries less technical sense and would be more familiar and revealing to most laypersons.

In short, *sexual problems, sexual dysfunctions,* or *sexual difficulties* are for the general description of the problems in sexual practice; *male impotence, erectile disturbance, erectile dysfunction* (ED), and *erectile difficulties* is specifically for describing the problems in initiating, maintaining, or sustaining an erection. So, **sexual difficulties** and **erectile difficulties** will be exclusively used. I hope the above discussion and clarification of the common terms for sexual issues be helpful for your future reading.

Sexual difficulties in men may range from the matters of the very "simple" to the "intricate" and "complex". Generally, *sexual difficulties* in men that are commonly encountered may be categorized into **three** groups: **erectile difficulties, disorders of desire (libido), ejaculation (premature or delayed),** and **orgasm**. Among these three, *erectile difficulties* is the most commonly experienced and mentioned. All these events may occur during the sexual interactions between the two partners, which are practiced by the majority of people. And those that are considered as deviant, abnormal, or unhealthy will be separately discussed in Part V.

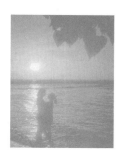

A lthough penile erection is the absolute necessity for sexual intercourse, any difficulty and frustration in sex life should be the matter of both parties, not just one.

16
Erectile Difficulties
– the Main Issue

Although *sexual difficulties in men* may appear in a wide range of presentations, ***erectile difficulties*** has been one of the centerpieces of attention among medical research, and care, over the last 30 years. Why? The answer is obvious: It is because **an erection, or no erection, from sexual arousal is the most visible, determining symbol of "potency" or "impotency" in mens' sex lives.** In fact, without a satisfactory erection, it would be impossible to have a vaginal penetration for sexual intercourse. As a result, there couldn't be the ability to procreate for the endless existence of human life. This fact should be enough to address the importance of a satisfactory erection.

As discussed in Part I, the value of sex life has evolved and expanded far beyond its primitive value of procreation since the ancient times. Today, in our contemporary sense, the contents of sexual activities have become a "routine" enjoyment, a mini-recreation, or a blessed gift from God in humans' daily life.

In ancient times, our life expectancy was as short as 30 to 45 years. Now, we can realistically expect a newborn to live more than 75 years on average. As we live longer in the ever-increasing complexity of our society, the natural aging process, and the unsurpassed amount of stress from daily chores, have made more and more men inevitably experience the frustration from no, or poor, erection. Such a frustration has increasingly demanded a solution; it is the "return" of their lost, or impaired, erection for sexual enjoyment and containment.

In sexuality for a man, no erection means no sexual intercourse and no chance to embrace the most intimate relationship of life and enjoy the peak of sexual pleasure. For a woman, without an erection of the clitoris (which is equivalent to men's penis), her sexual enjoyment through vaginal penetration is still possible as long as she is sexually aroused and wants to participate. This is the ultimate difference of sexual ability between men and women.

At a closer look, what can really be the problem with penile erection? Briefly speaking, it includes any difficulty that may prevent the penis from **timely and satisfactorily** vaginal penetration for sexual intercourse. The common conditions are: the penis could be not hard enough for vaginal penetration, or an erection can not be sustained long enough to complete a satisfactory intercourse, or a penis is too deformed to penetrate the vagina, such as a curved penis from Peyronie's disease.

After we realize the deserved respect for the care of men's erectile difficulties, let's move on to explore the magnitude of this issue.

In this section, let us focus on *erectile difficulty* (ED) in detail and continue our discussion with, ***"What is the key difference between men and women in their ultimate sexual expression?"*** The single most obvious difference in the ultimate sexual expression between men and women is the clearly visible *erection of the penis* from sexual arousal, which is functionally mandatory for sexual intercourse.

Beside this, men and women are very obvious in many forms. Externally, the natural genetic factors have made females very different from men in the ways they look. However, "superficial appearances" may be confusing in certain circumstances. For example, when you look at a person walking down a street, you may say in a surprise, "Heh! That person looks like a girl (or boy). What do you think?" But in fact, the reverse is true. Genetics! Sometimes a male's body appearance and behavioral expression is inclined more towards the feminine side. And conversely, sometimes, a female may possess certain attributes of a man's body appearance. And in "no way" does this genetic factor make either sex "less or more" of a person.

At birth, we differentiate male from female infants mainly by the appearance of their external genital organs. As we grow from infancy to childhood, adolescence to adulthood, Nature is continually at work making young males and females appear obviously more distinct and different toward their own unique gender appearance. *Breast enlargement and hip prominence of females after adolescence and puberty are the two most noticeable examples.* In addition, through natural evolution, humans' body hairs for protection and survival have faded away. Consequently, humans have to put on clothing to substitute the function of body hairs. In spite of these natural differences, the way we dress will often make these differences obscure, especially before adolescence. However, through millenniums of human existence, the fight for dominance and control of males over females has produced our current differences in traditional social function for both males and females. Almost all the aspects of human social functions have resulted from artificial man-made efforts; long hair, painted nails, dresses, pants, makeups, fashions, etc., are some of the stereotypes and mannerisms that separate the sexes.

In sexuality, according to the current value, the ultimate and obvious difference between men and women is evident in the appearance of penile and clitoral erection. Without an erected penis, natural copulation with sexual intercourse could not take place. Although the clitoris of females may be erect as well, it is not visually obvious. And through experience, it is usually sensed only at a close look or by a direct touch. For ultimate sexual intimacy, which would lead to sexual intercourse, a man cannot initiate the act without an erected penis. And, in spite of no real arousal and no erection of the clitoris, females are still able to participate (and even fake an orgasm if they want). **Because of these facts, the ability of penile erection has been the real emphasis and focus of concern in sexual difficulties in men**. Today, the inability to initiate, maintain, or sustain an erection to complete the acts of sexual intercourse is usually referred to as *male impotence, erectile disturbance*, or *erectile dysfunction* as just discussed above. For the problems of erection, *erectile difficulty* (ED) will be used for the reasons as just mentioned before. And from now on, I will focus on *erectile difficulty* (ED) which implies the difficulties in *initiating, maintaining*, or *sustaining* an erection to complete a mutually satisfied sexual intercourse.

How common are erectile difficulties?

The existing reports told us that the incidence for the occurrence of erectile difficulties varies by age and related diseased conditions. In general, it would be easy to remember it approximately as noted in the table below.

Age	30	40	50	60	70	80
% Impotence Rate	l	2	7	20	30	80

These figures indicate that the problem of sexual difficulties in men is much more common than that of cancer or heart disease. In considering the benefits of a satisfactory sex life to a man, his family, and even society, the care of sexual difficulties in men deserves due respect and a serious attention.

Unfortunately, in spite of its high prevalence and the availability of many treatment options, up to 30 million American men are having *erectile difficulties*, but less than two-third of them have ever been treated. Many men are uncertain, but there is one thing for certain, no man is alone if he has erectile difficulty. But sadly, many men are very reluctant to seek treatment ... and for many reasons: fear, disbelief, "machismo," alcoholism, a physical problem, mental dysfunction, adultery, and some men even believe that their sexual partners is the problem ... never the male.

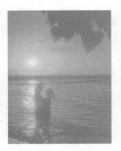

"What causes that?" (diagnosis) is the desirable product of teamwork of patient and medical professional, and is the pointer to treatment. But in reality, its accuracy is not always 100 per cent.

17

Common Causes of Erectile Difficulties

Up to some twenty or thirty years ago, most medical professionals and the general public still thought, and believed, that more than 80 to 90 percent of the time, erectile difficulties that men experienced during sexual performance were caused by mental conditions... it was purely in their heads (psychogenic). However, the latest findings from basic, and clinical, research over the last few decades have proven this type of belief to be faulty. In fact, it is now known that over fifty percent of the time, there are some types of physical conditions involved. Therefore, it is very important for both doctor and patient to pay equal attention to the issues affecting both mental and physical aspects of sexual functions and difficulties in the male patients.

To understand the subtlety and complexity of developing

sexual difficulties in men, let's look at how a disease would usually develop and what the possible progression of a patient's complaints would be.

In general, the symptoms of a diseased condition can be very elusive, especially at its early stage. The clinical picture of a disease (sexual or otherwise) may vary widely throughout the course of its development. At the very beginning, the degree or severity of the complaints and the frequency of the occurrence of a symptom may be very mild, atypical, and vague. Also, the findings from a physical examination by medical professionals may be very inconspicuous and inconclusive. During the early stage of a disease, it is difficult for anyone, either patients or medical professionals, to believe that there is anything really wrong in these patients. In a real life, this can be a frustrating clinical scenario in the medical "diagnostic" practice. Unfortunately, it is more often the "commonplace" and not the "exception."

But as the disease slowly progresses, the complaints of the patient and the findings of the doctor's physical examination will gradually become more obvious and more revealing. At such a time, medical professionals are more able to pinpoint what is wrong with his patient. However, to expedite a diagnosis, a patient needs to use his common sense and become aware of what his body is trying to reveal to him. Through "awareness and sensitivity", a patient will be able to feel and recognize any subtle changes from within.

Generally, as time goes by, the degree of difficulty and the frequency of sexual difficulties from erectile difficulties would be more obvious and significant as it increasingly affects a man's daily life. Due to the increasing presence of poor, or no, erection, a man may start to feel puzzled with uncertainty, frustration, low self-esteem, and a loss of his sexual partner in the end.

Any factors that may affect the mental comfort to perform and the physical fitness to act will cause erectile difficulties in men. The factor(s) involved may be psychogenic (mental) or organic (physical), single or multiple. And well known to us, both mental and physical conditions may interact. For easy understanding, they may be categorized into two major groups: **psychogenic (mental)** and **organic (physical) causes.**

Psychogenic (Mental) Causes:

As discussed in the section of *Simplified Dynamics of Sexual Performance* in Part III, a minimal degree of requirement for either mental comfort to perform or physical fitness to act is mandatory. If a man's mental comfort falls below its minimally required level, it will be certain to have poor, or no, erection for his intended ultimate sexual intimacy with sexual intercourse. Many factors can impair a man's mental comfort to perform. Personal discord, occupational or financial stresses, or guilt of adultery, even fear of sexually transmitted diseases, etc., are commonly identified as causes. As a result, he may experience loss of libido or fear of performance, which is **the ultimate pathway of mental difficulty.** And he fails to perform.

However, some mental causes responsible for sexual difficulties may be self-inflicted or self-imposed. They usually result from their own misunderstanding and misinterpretation of the sequence of events. But fortunately, it can be easily identified and corrected with common sense. There are two conditions that have not been uncommon to some men. To avoid such a misinterpretation, misunderstanding, and mismanagement of these two situations, it is worthwhile to share with you what I feel, think, and practice, and discuss them in detail as follows:

Incompatibility Between Mental Expectation and Physical Ability:

You may wonder why I place the situation of *incompatibility between mental expectation and physical ability* at the beginning of the discussion on mental causes for men's sexual difficulties. It is because even though it is not uncommon, it is frequently misunderstood. However, most times the anxiety or fear of performance resulting from this situation could be easily identified simply by self-awareness and is easily self-corrected. Therefore, a good understanding of this situation will help you walk out of the mess of this kind of sexual difficulty. To identify it, it is important to know the fact that an incompatible mental expectation is simply based on a misunderstanding of the natural working capacity of our mind and body. **Once properly recognized, it is easy for a man to dissolve, and thus resolve, the matter privately**.

It is true, and common, for a man to have his own stereotype of expectation to achieve a certain thing in life. The degree of expectation to do something successful, in general, is directly proportional to the degree of his past success and the importance in doing it. Achieving success in anything will make a man feel more secure, valuable, rewarded, and fulfilled than what he used to be. Such an experience in successfully doing something relaxing, cheering, fulfilling, and rewarding will naturally lead a man to repeat doing it over and over again in the future. Therefore, the higher the degree of success, the more intense such a tendency to achieve success will be. This recycling phenomenon of doing anything has been a predictable pattern of how a man behaves. As a matter of fact, this pattern of behavior is merely a primitive instinct of survival and is very similar among all species of animals. In other words, it represents a repeated process of reconditioning. This scenario of behavioral pattern is also specifically descriptive for a man to endlessly pursue his sexual pleasure in life. It becomes his motive to pursue an event of such a nature. He then has a desire to take actions to fulfill and enjoy it on his terms. However, Nature keeps all of the events in the universe changing and constantly moving. To Nature, such a change is a rule of life.

In Part III, I discussed the occurrence of such a change in the mental comfort to perform and the physical fitness to act as a result of aging. The memory of the glorious events in the past makes a man reluctant to give up what he has accomplished and possessed in life. Commonly, the medical world has noticed that many activities in life are related to an intentional struggle against the inevitable aging process. Let's take the intensity of exploring the methods of skin care as an example. To deceive the truth of one's age, many topical or systemic medications, and even surgical means to smooth the skin wrinkles from aging, have been in use. However, in the end, people who have received intense skin care still do not live longer than those without it. Fortunately, through the wisdom of Nature, most men and women are able to timely and graciously recognize it and adjust their lifestyles accordingly as they continue to work and enjoy their daily activities. However, unfortunately, such a gracious adjustment in life does not occur in some men and women. For example, the successful experience of sexual pleasure can make many men and women very reluctant to lessen their intensity, or their desire, to pursue sexual pleasure as their age advances. This situation has frequently produced a clinical situation of being incompatible between their mental comfort to perform and their physical fitness to act. Typically, a man almost always loves to retain his glorious memory of an intense sexual pleasure that was experienced at the peak of his highest level of sexual intimacy, usually through intercourse. But I must remind my readers and patients of being realistic and not to fix a standard so high that your mental expectation would easily exceed your own physical capacity. Bluntly speaking, physical capacity falls behind mental expectation. Naturally, a man may increasingly become more frequent and obvious in having various degree of failure during a high level of sexual intimacy – sexual intercourse. To remedy this situation, a man must make a timely adjustment to balance his mental comfort to perform and physical fitness to act or face more failures and frustrations in his future attempts.

Now, you may ask, "Is this because I am getting old?" In fact, yes, everyone does! However, getting older does not mean that you have give up, or withdraw from, all the enjoyment of sexual pleasure. In fact, many men of high age still retain their ability in erection and sexual intercourse. And yet, most men's erectile difficulties can be effectively managed and successfully rehabilitated with current concepts, practice and technology as long as their mental and physical conditions are allowable to perform and act.

At this time, it would beneficial for all men and women to understand some of the mental and physical changes that will inevitably take place during their aging process, which may directly or indirectly affect their sexual response and performance. The general direction of such an "aging change" follows a certain pattern. However, the degree and frequency of changes in individuals is not always the same although the male and female partners are at the same age. Keep in mind that at "all times" your quest for perfect sex must be followed. Remember that it is the pursuit of perfect sex, and not being perfect, that you strive to achieve.

What are the aging changes in sexual response and performance?

Sexual desire and performance of males are at their peak usually between the ages of 15 and 25 years . Afterwards, some noticeable changes in sexual response increasingly appear as men age. This process usually begins at ages 40 to 50, and will affect almost every mechanism and phase of humans' sexual response cycle. The changes may be slow and subtle from time to time. But, in fact, after 40, a man will take a longer time to achieve an erection and progress to the stage of orgasm and ejaculation during coitus. Meanwhile, erection, orgasm and ejaculation all occur with less force and intensity. Please also remember that the degree of these changes may vary in the same person from time to time. But, without a proper understanding of these facts and variations, many men may have some "personal" unrealistic expectation as well as for their sexual partner. Inevitably, one or both will experience some uncertainty and performance anxiety, which is the common pathway to affect a man's sexual performance.

The followings are four examples of noticeable changes in men's sexual responses that occur during aging, which I believe are important and worth our further discussion. And you will have a better understanding of reality in order to achieve the potential benefit of self-correction.

1. Prolonged refractory period:

Normally, every man would experience a period of time after orgasm and ejaculation during which he will be absolutely unable to respond to any mental and/or physical sexual stimulation to generate an erection. This period of time is called the *absolute refractory period of sexual response cycle.* Following this absolute refractory period, he will observe another period of time during which he becomes aware, only to some degree, of response to mental and physical stimulation with a subsequent erection. This period is called the *relative refractory period of sexual response cycle.* The duration of absolute or relative refractory period varies from person to person, and from time to time for even the same man. As the aging process advances, these refractory periods tend to become longer. Again, they vary among different men and at different times.

And to further realize these aging changes, let us think back in time to any sexual experiences you might have had as a youth. Do you remember when you were about 20 years old or so? At that age you were very resilient to sleep deprivation. You could stay up all night, or as late as you wanted to, and get up as early as you wanted to, and are still be able to put in a full day's work. In other words, you had a great amount of physical flexibility and mental reserve. However, as you have noticed, your physical and mental tolerance has slowly deteriorated as your age increased. A little lack of sleep now makes your mental and physical ability unable to satisfactorily complete tasks the same way as you used to in your youth.

And as for your sex life, you probably could remember the fact of the changes in your durability and recovery time after sexual intercourse. And at the age of 20 or so, within a matter of hours after orgasm and ejaculation, your desire for sexual intimacy could arise quickly and you were ready to conduct again another full course of successful sexual intimacy. But as your age increases, every thing needed for proper sexual functions now takes a longer period of time to recover. Then again, this is one of nature's little realities. Fortunately, many men have been able to wisely realize this and have realistically adjusted their expectations to comply with their physical durability and performance. By doing so, men will become happier in their sexual intimacies and, of course, in life as well.

How long are these periods supposed to be? As I just stated, they will vary from time to time and from man to man. In general, as age increases, such periods will gradually increase. If a man without proper knowledge or understanding of this fact tries to initiate an erection for sexual intercourse during these periods, he is doomed to a failing disappointment! An experience of this kind of "difficulty" clearly comes from himself due to his ignorance of sexual misunderstandings. Therefore, it is reasonable to state that the more a person understands the nature of the problem, the more effective one may work around any sexual difficulties, and accomplish more in his favor.

However, there will be times when a failure to achieve an erection may be due to an undue pressure, which may directly or indirectly come from the demand of a sexual partner. Specifically, if the male attempts to have sexual intercourse to please his sexual partner well before he has naturally recovered from completing a full course of sexual acts, he would most likely experience an inadequate performance in sexual intercourse. The full course of sexual acts covers all the phases normally and usually ranges from indirect foreplay, direct foreplay, excitement, erection, sexual inter-course, orgasm, ejaculation, resolution and, finally, a "full" recovery. Nevertheless, a man may try to please his sexual partner or show his sexual partner that he is really "mascu-line and able" in order to retain the continuation of their relationship. He then acts prematurely, fails, and then disap-points himself, and his sexual partner. This situation not only represents the fact that he acts prematurely, but also under undue anxiety about the relationship as well. This is also a good warning for any man to realize that there are reasons, one or multiple or in combination, for poor perfor-mance. Therefore, please understand and respect the reality of the problem and adjust any negative behaviors accord-ingly and naturally. **Life will be more fulfilling and hap-pier for any man if he knows when and how to adjust.**

2. Less psychogenic erection:

While a man is at his young age, say, at late teens or early 20's, many things can induce a sexual fantasy, such as a certain scent, a certain song, or a sensational photo, may be strong enough to initiate an instant erection. At times, that is why a young man might have experienced a social embar-rassment resulting from an unwanted, or untimely, erection while he walked around. The ability to achieve such an erection is known as *psychogenic erection*: a thought of some sexual content that can induce an erection.

As a man ages, he will progressively notice that he is be-coming less sensitive and responsive to a sexual fantasy. Eventually, he may not have any erection at all even while he is viewing some sensational pictures. Such an emerging, less responsiveness to mental stimulation is a natural change of aging; it does not mean that his ability to have an erection comes to an end. Instead, all what he does need in order to have an erection is more direct physical stimulation, especially to his penis from himself or his sexual partner.

Moreover, if you are at the stage of no more psychogenic erection, by no mean is your sexual ability completely lost. Instead, you just move onto another stage of reality of life and you are still able to perform sexually as long as you understand these changes, are patient, and possess a mental and physical readiness. In fact, it is not infrequent to see a man at his 80's or 90's who is still able to have an spontaneous erection if he has a good sexual desire and no physical difficulty exists to impair his erection.

3. A need for more physical stimulation and time to initiate erection:

How much of physical stimulation does a man need? Of course, it can vary from time to time as well as from person to person. Therefore, it is not advisable for men to compare their ability to achieve an erection with someone else's. Such a comparison may bring forth the feelings of anxiety or inferiority. And in turn, this situation will affect his sexual performance.

Although most men can usually provide direct physical stimulation to their penis, it is highly advisable that their loving and willing sexual partners participate in such physical stimulation. The participation of a sexual partner is usually indicative of the existence of a good interpersonal relationship, which, as discussed before, is the important part of the foundation for a healthy and meaningful sex life.

4. Delayed ejaculation:

As well, as I previously stated, the timing for orgasm and ejaculation will gradually slow down through aging. But please do not feel badly about it. It is normal and may actually be a blessing in disguise. Normal ability does slow down as a man ages. This may be a nature's precaution against heart and/or circulatory overload. Overall, your ability of heart, circulation, and overall physical tolerance will not act as well, or as fast, as when you were young.

Knowing these four unavoidable, yet expected, aging changes in sexual response and performance will help many men who have erectile difficulties correct themselves timely and regain their lost sexual ability peacefully and privately.

An Isolated or Sporadic Failure in Sexual Intercourse:

In life, no man is able to successfully perform a task 100% of the time. There will be times that a man may fail to complete a task and/or meet his personal goal. This is the reality of life and of human nature. However, if you occasionally fail to perform sexual intercourse as well as you might expect, **how are you going to deal with such an unpleasant experience?**

The occurrence of an isolated, or sporadic, failure in sexual performance is not uncommon to some men, young or old. Usually, it occurs at the time while they are drunk, over tired, or over anxious due to whatever the reasons are. In other words, it is while his mental and/or physical conditions are inadequate. However, generally, it would more frequently happen to elderly men because their span of physical flexibility narrows and weakens as their age increases. The reasons and dynamics of such a phenomenon are discussed in Part III.

1. What is the general significance of such an occurrence?

More or less, any form of sexual failure will produce some detrimental impact onto a man's ego and confidence. Subsequently, it will affect his mental comfort to perform during further attempts. In general, the degree of detrimental impact is directly proportional to his personal sense of the importance of his next attempt. And the higher the degree of importance, the worse the degree of anxiety, frustration, and even fear, will be. For example, if his inability to sexually perform may potentially lead to a discontinuation of an existing relationship with his sexual partner, then his anxiety and fear to anticipate a repeated failure will increase dramatically. As a result, inevitable failure is virtually predictable. It can be a self-fulfilling prophecy. And so he falls victim of performance anxiety.

As a reader of this book, or as a patient of mine, you might ask, "Is it possible for a man to overcome this difficult situation?" Of course it is, but only if he learns how to deal with it properly. And by continuing to read on, by understanding what the information is telling you, and by utilizing your newly founded information, you will begin to deal with your sexual difficulties most properly.

2. What should a man do after an occasional failure in his sexual performance?

I can predict that you will feel puzzled and embarrassed because you know that you didn't have any sexual problems before such a thing happened. Do not allow this situation to trouble you. Remain calm and please do not panic. Remember also that an occasional failure in sexual performance is nothing unusual in life; in fact, it even happens to some young men. You're not alone! Fortunately, this situation is usually correctable by itself if he possesses the knowledge of this reality and knows how to deal with it properly. The key solution is simple and clear; that is **"Don't panic, don't overreact to it and let the Nature do the work for you."**

You are already familiar with, and aware of, the dynamics of the interaction between the mental comfort to perform and the physical fitness to act as previously described. Therefore, it will not be difficult for you to honestly analyze what went wrong. Please read and truthfully answer the following:

1. *Are you still recovering from your last orgasm and ejaculation? Remember there is a duration called "refractory period" after orgasm and ejaculation, which is naturally expected for every man. Its duration varies from person to person and will become longer as you age.*

2. *Are there any seriously stressful conditions present in your life? Examples are medical illness, surgical recovery, passing of a loved one, monetary problems, physical exhaustion, etc.*

3. *Have any sexual failures occurred due to some sudden events such as heavy drinking, an overuse of a drug(s), a fight with someone, including your own sexual partner, a family member, a friend, or an acquaintance?*

4. *Has there been any potential personal, occupational, family, or financial crisis to distract your concentration from sexual performance?*

These situations are the common events in life that may alter your mental comfort to perform and your physical fitness to act to a level below its individual, or minimal, requirements. Through your personal and honest review of these events, if you suspect, or discover, one or more of these events has affected your mental comfort or physical fitness, clearly time itself will be your best friend and medication to effectively improve your ability. In addition, you would have to make some positive adjustment to deal with any personal or financial problems realistically. Meanwhile, be sure to resume and continue your daily activities as usual and enjoy your sex plays in the phase of indirect foreplay to assure a good interpersonal relationship with your sexual partner. When your physical condition is ready, you can progress to direct foreplay, intercourse, orgasm and ejaculation once again.

On the other hand, if you discover that your difficulties mainly result from one or more of these events, and it is affecting your mental comfort to perform, you would need to focus on the efforts to correct these identifiable, unfavorable conditions and improve them honestly with the program described. For more details on how to maximize success in your sex life, please refer to Part III.

However, over-anxiety and impatience may prematurely lead you to seek medical professionals before you need to. Keep in mind, as long as you are feeling and getting better day by day, you are advised to be patient to see what will be your eventual and optimal improvement. **"Time" is a very reasonable thing to consider and it is often the best medicine for you when healing is expected.** It is a part of our common sense in life. Again, time, nature, personal effort, and patience are your best friends to improve, and cure, your difficulties before unnecessarily seeking professional medical help.

However, if the difficulty continues for more than two or three months with no identifiable or perceivable progress from your efforts for self-improvement in spite of time, resting, nurturing, and faithfully practicing the art of perfect sex, I would then advise to seek active medical help.

Can psychological conditions affect your performance permanently? Yes, it is possible and is dependent upon your own coping ability in managing the stress from daily chores of realistic life. But it is extremely rare to be permanent. Your coping ability is the end-product of your life-long learning and is related with your social and cultural backgrounds and personal fantasies. Typically, erectile dysfunction from psychogenic (mental) causes is usually situational; that is usually associated with a specific time, a specific place, a specific sexual partner, or in any combination thereof. If the situation and the environment are right, you will respond well to sexual stimulation and you will have no problem to get a satisfactory erection for successful sexual intercourse. But if the situation and environment are not comfortable, sexual responses will negate any further involvement in sexual activity and/or intimacy.

With your understanding the reality of life and the importance to take care of daily personal chores and to cope with any undue stresses that probably result from your improper personal management, a timely recovery from an occasional failure can be anticipated.

However, sometimes your self-improvement with coping ability may not be enough. And you may fall into a mental trap called depression. To be aware of depression, please ask yourself if you are, or have been experiencing, the following: *Have you had any trouble falling asleep? Have you felt that you are not able to do anything without an effort. Have you always felt tired? Have you felt that you have lost appetite for food for no physical reason?*

All of these situations may suggest the presence of depression. To confirm the possibility of a major depression, please also think if you have a least five of the following conditions persisting for at least two weeks. They are;

1. depressed mood,
2. loss of interest or pleasure in all, or almost all, usual activities,
3. feelings of worthlessness, or excessive or inappropriate guilt,
4. diminished ability to think or concentrate, or indecisiveness,
5. fatigue or loss of energy,
6. insomnia or increased need for sleep,
7. feeling slowed down or restless and unable to sit still,
8. significant weight loss or weight gain, and
9. recurrent thoughts of death or suicide.

If you have any, or a combination, of the above conditions as described, please see a mental health professional for possible depression.

With this information, you can be alert so that you may have a timely appropriate medical attention and help. If so, the joint effort of medical professional and you can rescue your difficulty from mental depression and make your life up and running again.

Case Study: *JK, a 59 year old man complained of a decrease in sexual desire and poor erection at sexual attempt. History taking revealed his wife (46 years old) wished to have sexual intercourse four to five times per week and he was virtually only able to perform coitus at most two times a week. He clearly sensed the pressure from inside and outside himself. Through* **basic sex counseling**, *the pressure from incompatibility between mental expectation and physical ability was identified. A simple understanding and internal adjustment in the frequency of sexual intercourse solved the patient's sexual difficulties.*

Case Study: *AH, a 22 year old man complained of intermittent poor sexual performance over the weekend. History indicated that the patient wanted to have sexual intercourse four to five times over a weekend because the patient and his girlfriend were only able to get together over the weekend every two or three weeks. In his mind, their frequent sexual intercourse would be helpful to maintain their newly established relationship. And he became very anxious toward future sexual performance. After* **basic sex counseling**, *the patient and his girlfriend were able to realize the natural law of the dynamics between mental comfort to perform and physical fitness to act (see Section 8, page 47). And his sexual concerns resolved timely.*

These two examples are to show how an undue pressure from the inside and/or outside of the patient can affect a

man's sexual performance. Apparently, their poor performance results from the combination of unrealistic expectation, misunderstanding, and maladjustment of sex life. A good
understanding of such interactions can help, improve, and
solve many of men's sexual difficulties timely.

Organic (Physical) Causes:

As stated at the very beginning of this section, organic
causes have been found to contribute to men's erectile dysfunction in about fifty percent of cases. Also, from the understanding of the anatomy and function of male genital
organs, especially the penis, it would be not difficult for you
to imagine, and know, what may cause the penis to poorly
respond to mental and/or physical sexual stimulation. What
are they?

1. Vasculogenic Circulation
(Problems in circulation):

a. *Poor arterial circulation to the penis*

This condition is not uncommon, especially in elderly men.
It is usually caused by a partial, or a complete, obstruction
of the arteries that supply blood to the penis, usually resulting from the process of arterial blood vessel hardening,
known as *atherosclerosis,* or clot formation inside penile
arteries. This process is just like the obstruction of coronary
arteries supplying heart muscles. By far, it is the most common cause for poor circulation to the penis and is accountable for about 40% of men with erectile difficulties from a
physical reason. The end-result is a failure to adequately fill
up the spaces of sponge bodies inside the penis. Usually,
this condition is not surgically repairable. While a surgical

attempt to bypass the blockage may be undertaken, the long-term outcome has been poor.

In addition, any surgery, or trauma, in the pelvic area close to the prostate, bladder, and penis may cause a similar blockage resulting in an unwanted artificial interruption or diminished circulation to the penis. The common examples are radical prostate surgery (radical prostatectomy through lower abdomen or perineum, the area between scrotum and anus) for prostate cancer and colon/rectal surgery for rectal cancer. Similar problems resulting from trauma are pelvic fractures with or without injuries to the channel (urethra) or the prostate. This usually happens to the patients of a younger age. In selected cases of this kind, surgical attempt to bypass the traumatic blockage (penile revascularization) can be performed. This type of procedure has been observed to have about a five-year success rate with only a few complications in about 65% of cases. Therefore, the bypass procedure to re-establish a blood supply to the penis is worthwhile for this small group of men.

If the obstruction of blood supply to the penis is caused by atherosclerosis, the difficulty in getting an erection occurs slowly and progressively. As time goes by, it will become more evident. The degree of difficulty, in general, will be proportional to the degree of blood vessel obstruction. However, if it is caused by a surgery or trauma, the timing of the onset is sudden and coordinated with that of the related incidences. Therefore, a detailed medical history is a very important clue of the possible events concerning your sexual difficulties.

b. *Venous leakage or improper venous occlusion during the process of erection:*

Normally, while an erection occurs, the veins draining the

penis will be partially blocked in order to generate high blood pressure inside the sponge bodies of your penis so that an erection can be maintained and sustained for the completion of a sexual intercourse. But there is a time that such a required mechanism for venous occlusion fails to take effect. The end-result is a failure to effectively store the blood inside the penis. Clinically, the patients with this disease are usually still able to have a good erection at the beginning, but are not able to maintain and sustain it for completing intercourse. To confirm the existence of venous blood leakage, medical professionals need sophisticated equipment to measure the blood pressure inside the spongy bodies of the penis as well as to locate the sites of leakage. However, such equipment is not readily, and commonly, available for most practicing urologists. Also, the interpretations of these test results are not standardized.

For conservative treatment, a vacuum constriction device (VCD), or a heavy-duty rubber band, such as the one called Actis (venous flow controller) from Vivus, Inc., would be an effective conservative, yet practical, choice. For a definite treatment, an extensive exploration and ligation (tie off) "all" the veins draining the penis is required. Theoretically, it is an attractive and sound procedure. In reality, its long-term result has been far from satisfactory with a success rate of about 25 to 65% because of its later development of collateral circulation, which are new veins that form naturally to get around the blockage. Therefore, it is still considered to be experimental at most.

Recently, a specific muscle right onto the inner portion of the paired (2) corpora covernosa (page 28), called ischiocavernosus muscle as a part of pelvic floor muscles was found to have an effect to decrease or stop venous leakage.

A program of intense pelvic floor muscle exercise showed a favorable effect to control venous leakage and was reported as good as that from vein ligations. Therefore, it is worthwhile to practice such an exercise for the patients with suspected mild venous leakage.

2. Neurogenic Causes *(Diseases affecting the nerve system regulating erection):*

Erectile difficulty from neurogenic causes is due to nerve diseases such as degeneration, infection, inflammation, tumors, or injuries in peripheral nerves, specific parts of spinal cord, and the brain. Diabetes, uremia (severe kidney failure) and amyloidosis can affect peripheral autonomic nerve; this condition is frequently called *neuropathy*, such as diabetic neuropathy. In addition, radical surgery or radiation for controlling the cancers of prostate, bladder, colon or rectum may cause an injury to local peripheral nerves. All these conditions involving peripheral nerves may be associated with erectile difficulties in men. And the diseases involving spinal cord and spinal cord injuries by accident, surgery, disc herniation, tumors, or congenital spinal deformities, multiple sclerosis, tabes dorsalis (a form of syphilis) can cause erectile difficulties as well. Examples of brain diseases causing erectile difficulties are tumors, surgery, epilepsy, stroke, headache during sexual activities, Parkinson's disease, electrical brain therapy, etc. A detailed medical history will reveal a correlation between the onset of a change in sexual function and the disease itself.

The direct effect of all diseases affecting the nerve system will eventually impair the blood supply to the penis because the affected nerves become unable to relate the message of sexual stimulation properly. As a result, the smooth muscles of blood vessels and sponge bodies fail to relax normally and the ability to gain an erection is impaired or failed. Subsequently, an erection cannot be fully initiated and/or maintained. This situation may also have an overall effect on the well-being and mental health of patients, spouses, and/or sexual partners because of the impact from treatment, medication, physical inconvenience, depression, etc.

3. Diabetes Mellitus and Other Endocrine (Hormonal) or Metabolic Disorders:

Diabetes mellitus is by far the most common chronic illness caused by a hormone deficiency. Its process will eventually produce a wide range of adverse effects in the body. If the blood sugar level is not closely regulated, many of its victims will develop an acute illness from metabolic abnormalities. The worst of these is diabetic coma. As the disease progresses, sooner or later, it can produce some chronic adverse effects in the nervous system (diabetic neuropathy), arterial blood vessel hardening (arteriosclerosis), and damage to kidneys (diabetic nephropathy), etc. As a result, erectile difficulties have occurred in as high as 60% of diabetic men reporting to be impotent. And it is responsible for about 30% of all physical causes for male erectile difficulties.

Please note that the degree of complications and effects associated with diabetes is highly connected to the duration and control of the disease. As expected, either acute or chronic adverse effects from diabetes mellitus can affect a man's physical fitness to act and/or mental comfort to perform.

In my medical practice, there have been times when male patients come to me stressing their difficulties in achieving a good erection. Through a careful historical and a medical evaluation, it is not infrequent to discover that some of them have diabetes mellitus without any prior history of the disease; proving that no one should ever take anything for granted.

4. Low Male Hormone (Testosterone):

The male hormone, *testosterone*, is well known and essential for the development and maintenance of manhood. If its blood level is "too" low, a man's sexual desire can be impaired. In life, as a man gets older, his blood level of testosterone tends to become lower as well. However, the blood level of testosterone does not necessarily reflect the real effect of this hormone in the body. In fact, in an otherwise healthy man with a normal sexual desire, the possibility of having a deficiency in testosterone is not likely. And low male hormone is only responsible for less than 3% of all physical causes for erectile difficulties or impotence. However, the use of male hormone has been common, and even excessive, due to easy access to it from many medical offices. A prescription of testosterone will make patients feel good about themselves, as well as their physicians, mainly from the so-called placebo effect of any "drug", and the feeling he might perceive that he has been kindly cared for.

In practice, if a man is found to have a low, or relatively low, level of testosterone, a trial use of testosterone for one month is reasonable.

Others ,such as the overproduction of prolactin or some hormones of the adrenal glands and the underproduction of thyroid hormones have been observed, and blamed, for causing male erectile difficulties. Fortunately, these hormonal dysfunctions are not common and they can be suspected by taking a medical and sexual history and performing a physical examination carefully.

5. A Host of Acute and Chronic Illnesses:

The symptoms of an acute illness can greatly diminish a patient's sexual desire because his mind is so preoccupied by the ill feelings of severe pain, nausea, vomiting and weakness. Acute abdominal operations, a painful back sprain, severe arthritis, and being in a plaster cast for extremity or spinal fractures are common examples.

But understandably, sexual difficulties resulting from an acute illness are usually temporary. Fortunately, time and Nature will "cure" you if you are not adversely affected by a failure in sexual performance as those conditions described in this section, *Psychogenic (Mental) Causes,* (page 98).

At times, physical disability and disfiguration from chronic illnesses may also produce direct, and indirect, effects on a man's mental comfort to perform and physical fitness to act. And while under such chronic conditions, the effects on sexual difficulties may be more complicated and lingering. Thus, any medical professional or home-care and nursing for these will require a high level of skill and experience. And for the patients and families, the understanding, and the practice, of the basics (as described in Part III) are always useful and needed. But I strongly advise patients and families to work cooperatively with their medical professionals.

Any patient with a painful back sprain, severe arthritis, paralysis, in a plaster cast, after leg amputation, chronic kidney failure, chronic liver disease, various cancer diseases and anyone on chemotherapy are but few sampled victims suffering from the effects of their chronic diseases.

6. Medications:

Many drugs can cause a variety of sexual difficulties such as a decrease in sexual desire, an alteration in male hormone level, nerve control, or blood supply to the penis, and a change in the direction of ejaculation. Through these effects, the drugs may interfere with erection and ejaculation. Statistical information has shown that about 10 - 25% of all organic impotences are caused by the side effects of medication. As many as 275 drugs have been noted to adversely affect the ability of erection. Usually, the drugs involved are those used for treating high blood pressure, sleeplessness, anxiety, agitation, and depression. It is sure more drugs will be blamed for causing erectile difficulties (ED) as more medications will be discovered and used for these diseases. The number of drugs that cause sexual difficulties are so great that there is probably no medical professional that can really tell any individual (with 100% certainty) which drug(s), to what extent, will produce such side effects. Therefore, whenever the medications for these diseases are prescribed, only a general warning for potential side effects can be issued to the patients. However, no medical professionals can predict if such side effects will happen to an individual patient or not. In my practice, I just generally advise my patients to use the drugs as prescribed, but to closely watch for any side effects and/or abnormalities in their mental and physical well-being. And the moment they believe something is wrong after using medication, I strongly urge them to stop the drug(s) and immediately contact me. Therefore, it is a sound and reasonable advice for you to do the same.

The names of some common drugs with the side effects that cause sexual difficulties are alcohol, marijuana, LSD, Cocaine, Amphetamines, Methadone, Morphine, Heroin,

Inderal, Lithium, Valium, Halodol, Elavil, Tofranil, Mthyldopa, Clonidine, Reserpine, just to name a few common ones.

7. The Conditions Directly Affecting the Penis:

- Some of *congenital deformities* of the penis may be so severe that a successful surgical correction is impossible. Consequently, the penis is inadequate for sexual intercourse. In general, it is very rare.

- **Peyronie's diseases** is a disease that causes severe thickening and hardening of a part of the sheaths, usually of corpora cavernosa, from an unclear reason. The result is a curved penis at erection, which may be so severe that a vaginal penetration becomes impossible. At times, the patient may feel painful when his penis is erect.

- **Priapism** is a diseased condition of prolonged unwanted erection, which produces a state of high pressure and low oxygen level inside the sponge bodies of the penis for an undue long period of time. Its effect is painful erection. As a result, late permanent tissue damage with the scarring of the sponge bodies occurs, which will make a further erection impossible in about fifty percent of the patients. Priapism is not a result of normal sexual stimulation in any way. Instead, it may be related with the presence of sickle cell disease, trauma, leukemia, and certain medications. However, at present, priapism is most commonly caused by penile self-injection that is a frequently used option for treating erectile difficulties.

8. Miscellaneous Conditions that May Affect Maintaining and Sustaining an Erection:

A serious, and treatable, cause to affect erection is a mental distraction from an unbearable pain that appears during intercourse or toward the moment of orgasm and ejaculation. This condition is not commonly mentioned in medical practice. Nonetheless, they were experienced in the Author's practice. It is worthwhile to note their existence. Such a pain may occur sometimes after vasectomy, inguinal hernia repair, or in patients who have disc hernia or lower backache. Please do not get panic with such occurrences from these common medical conditions. After all, it is not common at all, but it does happen occasionally. It is the reality of consequence from an illness and life. If such a condition is suspected and could be verified, the underlying reason has to be treated as a definite care if the patient wants to have his erectile difficulty from such an unbearable pain restored. For the individual details, please always discuss the involved issue openly and honestly with your own medical professionals timely. To illustrate such an effect, I have a personal case for your review.

Case profile:

J. P., 63-years gentleman, visited me for his inability to maintain erection because of an unbearable pain at left groin region. A detailed history revealed that he was able to initiate a good erection as usual, but unable to maintain and sustain the good erection because of severe pain at left groin region while he was penetrating the vagina. And it was also noted that his erectile difficulty occurred about one month after left inguinal hernia repair somewhere and got worse as time went by. At his visit to me, it was about six months after his hernial surgery. In physical examination, a small severe tender spot near the inner end of inguinal incision was palpated. A "nerve block" was given to that special spot and the tenderness instantly disappeared. After three nerve blocks, the symptoms improved by about 45% in the patient's own words, but not sufficient enough to eliminate the pain and he still experienced mental distraction from the pain and inability to maintain and sustain erection for completing sexual intercourse. Eventually the suspected spot in the incision was explored, identified, and excised. As a result, his distracting pain disappeared and his erectile difficulty restored. And he returned to his missed wonderland of sex life and is a happy man again.

It is impossible for me to mention all the causes for erectile difficulties (ED) that result from a wide variety of diseases, operations, injuries, medications, and performance anxiety. Also, please do not feel scared and frightened by knowing so many causes for ED. Remember, knowledge is power. Correct knowledge can help you have the most reasonable option of care.

*M*edical care is not just for "I would rather be safe than sorry," but for practical need; common sense is the base of it.

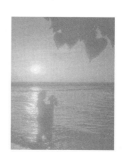

18

Evaluation of Erectile Difficulties

When a man experiences a difficulty to get an erection, naturally he may frustrate and become anxious. Unfortunately, as stated before, less than two-third of men with sexual difficulty due to no or poor erection have ever been evaluated and treated medically. However, when he does seek a medical help, it is his best interest to know when, what, and how he will be evaluated.

When Do You Need Help from Medical Professionals?

For your understanding, I have so far shared the ideas with you about the "real" value and respect of sex life, the theory and the practice of perfecting a satisfying sex life, and the causes for sexual difficulties in men from *erectile difficulties*.

The approach and methods described are both ideal and practical for initiating, developing, maintaining, and sustaining "perfect sex" for you and your sexual partner. Much of the resulting happiness from perfecting your sex life will significantly enrich the quality of your life. Accordingly, I hope that you will be able to utilize most, if not all, the advice and information that I have offered.

Now, let us assume, for one reason or another, that you are experiencing some difficulties in achieving a satisfactory sex life for your sexual partner and/or yourself. Naturally, you may desire to look for medical help and advice after you have understood and followed the approaches described in this book and still failed to satisfactorily improve your difficulties in a timely manner.

Living together in peace and harmony is one of the important things that we would like to do as a society and as individuals. And when a couple lives together in an intimate relationship, "peace and harmony" become especially important for perfecting a sexual life together. Therefore, when sexual difficulties arise and appear to be a contributing factor for the deterioration of a relationship, I would personally advise both partners to seek professional help as quickly as possible... do not wait for more than two or three months. But if you and your sexual partner have followed what I previously stated in the book, both of you will have little difficulty in maintaining a sound "interpersonal relationship" (indirect foreplay) to maximize "self-improvement" techniques. And from this point on, cooperatively decide when, where, and from whom you should seek medical help. However, once again, please do not wait for more than 2-3 months.

Now you are on the way to seek medical help. To be cost-effective in medical care, it is a good idea for you to be knowledgeable about the roles, responsibilities, and approaches that the medical professionals should provide for you, and how you can cooperate with them to maximize the benefits from their care.

Steps of Evaluation for Erectile Difficulties:

To achieve that goal, I am providing the following as a detailed, and concise, method of evaluation to reasonably confirm the underlying cause, or causes, for sexual difficulties. For a meaningful and intimate sex life involving two parties, it will require the devotion of time and effort from both parties through a cooperating and coordinating discipline of total sharing. And, in order to achieve the optimal benefits from professional care, the following steps should be completed in a timely manner. They are as follows:

a. *a cooperating and coordinating team involving you, your sexual partner, and medical professionals must be formed.*

b. *a detailed medical history about your general health and your sexual health should be obtained.*

c. *a detailed physical examination including external genital organs and prostate must be done.*

d. *some specific blood tests or other tests may be required.*

e. *a joint and reasonable decision on the method of care will be reached and provided.*

f. *a reasonable schedule for follow-up is needed.*

Now that you have a medical outline to follow, you will know what to expect down the road. Although you may experience some minor variations in the steps and procedures of care from different professionals, in general, such a range of coverage is effective and reasonable. At least, that is how I have conducted my successful medical practice throughout the years.

Below, I am going to go into greater detail for each step outlined:

a. Form a Good Team.

As I stated before, our traditional view of a man's sex life has delayed many men from seeking the help of medical professionals. But now, after reading the prior sections, I hope that such reluctance should be eased and resolved. You need to know that what you are doing is for the good of your sexual partner, your family, society, and not just for you alone. Although your sexual partner may be too "shy" to go to a medical office with you on the first visit, it is imperative that both of you and your medical professionals all meet, understand, and work together efficiently. A willingness to see medical professionals together usually suggests that there is a good interpersonal relationship between a couple. A well cooperating and coordinated team is the foundation of further work for you.

b. History Taking:

1. General Medical History:

The work of obtaining a general medical history will allow medical professionals to have a reasonable idea about your general medical and mental health, along with your educational, occupational, personal, social, and family background. However, you may be wondering, "How is all of this information obtained and what will my doctor do with it?" Although it is ideal to get this done directly by medical professionals, today it is not uncommon to have medical allied professionals such as trained nurses, physician assistants, medical students, or residents initially screen the patient with a set of questions. Later, the medical doctor, usually the urologist in charge, will review and confirm the information that was just obtained from you (and, if available, your sexual partner).

"What questions are usually asked?" Most of you should be quite familiar with the questions if you have ever seen a doctor. Although there is usually a long list of questions, please read and review the following questions so that you will be prepared:

- *What is your marriage status?*
- *What is the extent of your education?*
- *What is your past and present occupation?*
- *What, and how, is your mental and physical stability now compared to then?*
- *Do you now have any problems with your heart, lungs, kidneys, liver, and brain?*
- *Have you ever been told in the past that you have a significant problem with your heart, lungs, kidneys, liver, brain, and/or circulation?*
- *Were you told that you have a diabetic disease? If yes, how has it been treated?*
- *What is your general attitude for dealing and coping with difficulty, frustration, or a failure in life?*
- *Are you allergic to any medication?*

- *Are you recently, or presently, taking any medication? If yes, for how long and for what reason? Also, please list the medications and their dosage as complete as possible.*

- *What is your priority in your physical, mental, financial, personal, and family life?*

- *How often do you experience depression?*

- *Do you have any hobbies? If so, what are they?*

- *What do you do to relax?*

- *Do you have a healthy relationship with your sexual partner?*

All the above information will allow your medical professional to have a reasonable understanding about your needs. Your doctor will be able to discuss with you the proper procedures and actions that will help you.

2. Sexual History Taking:

This part of your medical history is usually obtained in a similar fashion as general medical history was taken and for the same reasons. However, in this session of history taking, your doctor will be more direct and ask you more detailed questions about your sex life, so please be open and honest. I personally would like to cover the following questions:

- *Describe as best as you can what your sexual concern is.*

- *When did you first notice there was a problem in your sex life? And if your sexual difficulties have existed for a long period of time, why did you delay in seeking professional, medical help?*

- *Did your problem happen to you suddenly or slowly? If slowly, I will need to know if your problem or condition progressively worsened? If suddenly, I will need to know if there was any incident or event that might have precipitated or prompted your difficulties.*

- *Do you still get a good morning erection when you wake?*

- *Are you still able to achieve a good erection, off and on, under different situations such as a thought fantasy of a potential sexual partner or the viewing of an erotic graphic movies/pictures?*

- *When you develop a good erection, do you have any problem maintaining or sustaining it?*

- *Did you have some disturbing or distracting thoughts in your mind while you attempted to have sexual intimacy and intercourse? If so, please let me know what they are?*

- *How often do you like to have sexual intercourse while you were satisfied with your sex life?*

- *How often do you like to have sexual intercourse now? Why?*

- *When did you last have a normal erection?*

- *When did you last have sexual intercourse?*

- *On a scale of 1 to 10, how would you compare your present ability to have an erection with the past when you were 100% satisfied with your erections?*

- *When did you have your last vaginal penetration? What was the degree of erection then on a scale of 1 to 10 (10 being highest)?*

- *Did you have any premature ejaculation or any difficulty in maintaining or sustaining your erection to complete intercourse?*

- *What is your sexual desire now compared to then?*

- *Who is your sexual partner? How long?*

- *Please tell me about the age, health, personal life, and sexual desire for intercourse of your sexual partner.*

- *Does your sexual partner enjoy sexual intercourse? Does she usually have an orgasm? If yes, how many times out of ten times did she experience orgasm?*

- *Does your sexual partner usually give you sufficient physical stimulation to your penis and/or other desire-arousal parts of your body?*

- *Do you directly or indirectly sense that you sexual partner is not satisfied with your sexual performance? If yes, how does your sexual partner express it?*

- *Do your sexual partner empathize with your sexual problems and difficulties?*

- *The final question that your urologist might ask is, "As your doctor, What would you like me to do for you right now?"*

After acquiring all the above information, your medical professional will have a better understanding of your sexual difficulties. So far, knowing and understanding why it is important to work with your medical professional is extremely important to bring about proper help to your situation and condition.

What is next? It is the basic discipline in medicine to have a good history and a physical examination. Now, let us proceed to explain the procedures of a thorough physical examination.

c. Physical Examination:

During this step of your care, your medical professional will thoroughly examine you by what he/she can see, physically touch, hear, and monitor. Routinely, I need to check out your heart to discover if there is any murmur, irregular beat, or enlargement. Also, I have to know if your lungs are clear and ventilating well for you, if your external genital organs and prostate are in good shape, and if your pulse, blood pressure, lymph nodes, nervous system, etc. are all right.

All the above steps can be completed during your first visit. Your medical professional will have further impressions of what he/she can, and will, do for you, with your permission, of course, after the examination.

And after completing your physical examination, some tests will be taken to understand, or confirm, the impression (or convictions) that your medical professional has about your sexual difficulties. Some of these tests are basic and essential; others may be optional. Although the optional tests may enlighten your doctor's convictions under certain indications, they may be used simply for insurance or medicolegal purposes during possible future litigation or investigation, or even for financial reason. Whatever the tests are used for, make sure that you properly and reasonably understand why you are taking them and how they will be used to help you for the diagnosis and treatment of your sexual difficulties.

d. Basic Blood Tests:

Since most of my patients already have their own family doctors, I am usually able to have the result of some needed tests from other medical offices. Such an effort will allow me to know more about your health. Remember, in doing so, the repetition of testing can be avoided and the cost of care will be less and contained.

Now, let us assume you have been cared for under a family doctor and you come to see me, a urologist, for a personal sexual problem that deals with your inability to have an erection. The following are the specific tests that I would need to do for you in order to further understand your problem.

- *Fasting blood sugar:*

This test is to confirm if you are diabetic, or to check the level of your current diabetic control if you have been diagnosed as diabetic.

- *Blood tests for prostate specific antigen (PSA) and testosterone:*

Blood testosterone is done routinely for all men with low sexual desire (loss of libido), and/or small, soft testes. However, if a man is 45 or older and/or if he has abnormal finding in his prostate on digital rectal examination (DRE), I would do both testosterone and PSA at the same time. Why? It is because I would prescribe testosterone supplement for him at least on a trial basis if blood testosterone is low and clinically significant and there is no suspicion for prostate cancer.

Of note, an elevated PSA and/or any abnormal finding in the prostate from DRE are indicative of suspecting prostate cancer. And, a supplemental use of testosterone can accelerate its growth. Therefore, any men with elevated PSA and/ or any abnormal finding on the prostate from rectal examination should have further evaluation to confirm no high suspicion of prostate cancer before using any forms of testosterone.

The details of clinical significance of PSA, testosterone, and DRE may be difficult for most people to understand. To avoid unnecessary misunderstanding, please check with your own medical professional if you may have any related questions.

e. More Blood Tests:

The examples of more blood tests are tests for **prolactin, luteinizing hormone (LH), and follicular stimulating hormone (FSH).** The practical value for a routine use of these tests is debatable and controversial. But they are desirable for impotent men with low blood testosterone and loss of sexual desire. In my practice, I only used them very selectively. But for the details of their usage, again, please ask and check with your own medical professional when these tests are ordered. Please believe me, the complexity of interaction and implication among all these tests are beyond a real understanding of most people and the general public. Therefore, please do not let these tests bother and/or confuse you.

f. Nocturnal Penile Erection:

The research of penile erection at night, over an average sleep of 8 hours, has shown that the penis of normal potent men will have 3 to 5 episodes of a good erection. Penile erection usually occurs in about 25% of the total sleeping time, and each episode of erection will last about 20 - 30 minutes. Interestingly, penile erection is correlated well with the so-called periods of rapid eye movement (REM) of normal sleep. Based on this information, studies have documented the degree of nighttime erection to be the best test available today to see if a man's impotence is organic (physical) or psychogenic (mental) in origin. But the simplest test that a urologist may use is called snap-gauge. It is a device that is put onto the base of the penis at night for measuring the degree of penile erection. For a similar documentation, a sophisticated electronic device may be used in a special laboratory or at home. Please be aware, the test with an electronic device is expensive and could be unnecessarily overused for financial reasons.

If you have a poor nighttime erection as shown in the test, it indicates that you have an erectile problem from one or more physical causes. On the other hand, if you have a good nighttime erection, as shown by the test, it indicates that your problem is psychogenic (mental). The test results are indicating what, mental or physical, has played a major role to cause your poor erection.

Please remember that both organic and psychogenic factors usually interact to influence the overall quality of penile erection and sexual performance. At times, this test is only important for insurance companies; therefore it is not practically needed because a detailed history will be enough to indicate a mental or physical reason for a poor erection. However, this test will most definitely indicate a mental or physical reason for a poor, or no, erection.

g. CAT scan or MRI (special X-Ray examination) of the brain to rule out pituitary tumor:

It is rarely needed and is usually reserved for the patients with low blood testosterone, high blood prolactin, loss of libido, etc. Usually, these patients may have some other symptoms or signs such as headache or a change in vision. But again, please ask and check with your own medical professional if this test is ordered. I will not elaborate on them any further because the depth of such a description is beyond the scope and sequence of the purpose intended for this book.

h. Special Tests for Nerve Function and Blood Circulation to the Penis:

These tests are used more for the interest of investigation and research rather than for their practical use in the daily care of sexual difficulties. Also, they are usually only available in referral centers. Again, please ask and check with your own medical professional to find out why these tests are ordered. Again, I will not elaborate on them any further because further description of these tests are truly beyond the original purposes of this book.

Now, you have gone through the whole process of evaluation. However, in reality, a perfect set of evaluation remains to be seen or unknown. At best, all the evaluation that you have received might have been only reasonable. As the medical experiences in the filed of caring erectile difficulties (ED) are further accumulated and scrutinized, the sequence and amount of evaluation will surely be modified in order to reach the common goal of cost-effectiveness in today's medical care the duty that we, the people, should bear.

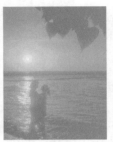

The best is most pleasing and attractive to hear but not true. No treatment option can rehabilitate an impaired sexual function from all causes for all men. The truth is none of treatment options is best, but, at most, most reasonable.

19
Treatment Options for Male Erectile Difficulties

General Consideration:

1. What Can, and Will, the Medical Profession Do for Your Health?

In general, the mission of medical professionals (physicians) is to use the current available knowledge, technology, and skills in their medical field **to make your whole body work as normal and as long as possible.** In other words, doctors work to rehabilitate patients back to their age-adjusted normal health and condition... nothing more, nothing less. I used to joke with my patients by saying, "I am a physician, not a magician. There is a limit on what I can do for you." Please do not get disappointed. Medical professionals can do a lot for you. Good examples are the medical advancements in the care of heart diseases, hip disability, kidney failure, sexual difficulties in men, and much more.

2. What Can, and Will, a Medical Professional (Usually a Urologist) Do for Your Sexual Difficulties?

What a urologist can do for your sexual difficulties is, simply stated, SEXUAL REHABILITATION. A urologist will utilize the current available knowledge, technology, and skills in this special field to investigate, diagnose, and treat the problems of your sexual difficulties. Allowing you to function as normal, and as long of a period of time as nature allows. That is your medical professional's mission to you.

3. When Will a Treatment Be Started?

There is no need to wait until all of the tests are completed before a treatment option is provided. The timing of the treatment should correlate with a practical need, understanding, and consideration of the "time", cost, commitment, and treatment that will be needed for your rehabilitation. Also, a period of time will be needed for a "true healing", and to allow for the least amount of stress upon your relationship. By the way, a consideration of cost-effectiveness in medical care by medical professionals and patients would be very much appreciated by all of us in society.

4. What Do You Need to Bear in Mind, and Be Ready for, before Any Treatment is Implemented?

As stated in Parts I and III, it is important for you to realize that the purpose of your ongoing sexual rehabilitation is to enrich the quality and quantity of life for you and your sexual partner. Also, it is equally important to be sure that your mental comfort to perform and your physical fitness to act are ready. Without such thought and practice for your sexual rehabilitation, the treatment that you receive will probably do very little for you and your sexual partner for a long-term basis. This is not a doctrine, it is a truth and a reality. I want you to be sure what your medical professionals (or a urologist) can do for you is really what you need, not just what you want or what a medical professional may say they can do.

5. What Kind of Treatment Option Will Meet Your Practical Need?

It is a good idea to start out with a treatment option of the least invasion and cost. Somehow, it has been noted that the treatment for sexual difficulties in men follows a similar path, no matter what the underlying cause for the sexual difficulties is.

In general, based on this formula, I divide the treatment options into five levels. They are; **Level 0** – no (or expectant) treatment, **Level 1** – basic sex counseling, **Level 2** – medications of less invasion, **Level 3** – assisted erection with mild invasiveness, and **Level 4** – implantation of penile prosthesis as the last resort for an active sexual rehabilitation. All of the options will be explained in greater detail. Again, please be sure that the treatment you will receive is to meet your practical need.

Treatment Options:

After reviewing the ideas on how to decide what kind of treatment option you really need in a practical and yet realistic term, let us look into what is the reasonable treatment option for your erectile difficulty.

Of note, the following discussion on the listed treatment options is not intended to cover *all* options and all their details. It represents the current logical and practical approach with high cost-effectiveness that the Author believes in. Also, the options and the sequence of their use may change from time to time. Therefore, an update may be made in the future edition to meet the current trend of practice.

Level 0: No (or Expectant) Treatment

No treatment?! A joke? No, it is not a joke. Yet, at times, it becomes a reality. I know this advice is not attractive and popular to some people; it is not what most patients want to hear when they are seeking a "cure" for their sexual difficulties. Furthermore, I hope you would not feel offended by this option of "no treatment". You may not agree with this option, but practical medical care should be directed toward improving the quality and quantity of life. And if the mental and physical readiness is not there due to a serious illness in the lungs or heart, the option of "no treatment" would be the most reasonable, probably the best, option for the patient at the time.

In the past, I saw a man at his 80's with erectile difficulty as well as severe chronic obstructive pulmonary disease (COPD or severe lung disease). Because of a severe loss of lung capacity, he needed a constant use of an oxygen (02) supplement for him to move around. At my office, he even fell into sleep within a few minutes after I turned around to complete his medical record. In other words, he is barely kept alive. However, he still wished to have an implantation of penile prosthesis because he had viewed a number of television programs showing what medical experts could do for men with impotence. Facing such similar clinical situations as a medical professional, I had to be honest and sure that what I did was for the practical need, and best interest, of my patients, not just for my professional satisfaction or moneymaking. Similar examples requiring no treatment are severe heart disease, severe depression, etc. Basically, for any man who is terminally ill or severely disabled from a disease and its treatment, I would recommend expectant treatment with comfort and encouragement for him to spend more valuable time with family, relatives or friends.

However, I have occasionally had patients who were severely or terminally ill, and they stated that they would rather have a few moments of fun with sexual intercourse than living a life without it. To my sensitive and sympathetic side, it makes sense. But from a more practical view and respect for life, as we observe today, I am not quite sure that they really wanted to die from having intercourse as opposed to living longer with their family. Fortunately, they changed their minds and did not undergo a penile implant. For a while, they were frustrated, but later, after an extended discussion and explanation, they realized that "no treatment" was their most reasonable choice.

Level 1: Basic Sex Counseling

In this session of sex counseling, I will review the following as discussed previously in Part III. To fulfill the basic natural pattern of a normal sex life, and to comprehend the expected changes from our inevitable aging, "understanding" is the key to an active and successful sexual rehabilitation. A full course of sex life itself represents a process of very heavy mental and physical drainage. A fulfilling sex life involves all the mental and physical activities in each phase of the sexual cycle that includes indirect foreplay, direct foreplay, sexual intercourse, orgasm, and ejaculation to resolution and recovery.

Whenever you wish to have sexual intercourse, it is wise and advisable to be sure that you are mentally comfortable to perform and physically fit to act. Also, be aware that your upcoming, ultimate sexual intimacy will not only enhance the quality and quantity of your life, but also that of your sexual partner. In other words, you need to be sure while having intercourse that you are not doing it under any mental and/or physical stress. . . for the "act" itself will be draining. Also, to fully understand the basic psychological aspects of sexuality, please review the discussions in Part I and III. But for now, I will need to reiterate some of the discussions.

An occasional failure in sexual intercourse can happen to any man, even at a very young age. Realizing this fact can be very helpful for you to resolve any frustration from such a failure and effectively recover in a timely fashion.

By now, you know that any act in life is an end product of the combination of your mental comfort to perform and your physical fitness to act. Aging can make a significant change in all kind of activities in life. For sexual activities, some of these changes are still mysterious and puzzling to many men. Why? They just tend to resist, and even resent, the appearance of these changes. Worst of all, some men do not even believe that such changes are happening to them. They simply continue their fantasy of "I am as young as I think," or "I am as good today as when I was 20 years old." These comments are not intended to discourage any man's ambition. Instead, I simply need to remind you of the upcoming, and unavoidable, changes in life as a result of aging.

And as you probably would agree, the more realistically a person can understand Nature, the more effectively a person can deal with the inevitable. Anyone can overcome the difficulties in life if they faithfully confront them. This simple understanding will work very well for your sexual rehabilitation. It will make you successfully continue along with your adventuring path toward the wonderland of "perfect sex".

Through my lifelong experience in medical practice, I have noted some discouraging situations that you would not like to have but may ultimately have to confront. Here I would like to share them with you as a precaution while you are seeking a medical care (for whatever the reason). What I say is not to berate the medical profession. Instead, what I am sincerely hoping for it is that you will have the best, honest environment of medical care. Through a general awareness of such an existence, all people from all different groups in society may work together for the best interest of all of us. And as you know, medical professionals are just human. They have to make a living and pay their bills as anyone else does. But the balance of power between patients and medical professionals is not equal. Usually, more or less, you are very anxious about your health and you need help. Under these stressful circumstances, you are mentally vulnerable and at a disadvantage. It is a common situation for patients to accept almost anything that medical professional would offer you without question and hesitation, especially when medical professionals are very courteous, sympathetic, and responsive to your demands.

Also, our traditional impression about medical professionals makes most people believe that all of them are generally

honest and respectful. Such an impression toward a professional will blind your common sense of what a medical professional will do for you. Please understand, I do not want
you to mistrust your medical professionals. In fact, fortunately, most medical professionals are still very decent, honest, and capable.

However, there may be times when you may confront some
uneasy situations that make you wonder why Dr. So an So
wanted you to come to his office so frequently for visits,
injection, tests, etc., over and over without seeing much
progress in the care of your condition. As you know, there
are a number of so-called GRAY AREAS (unknown or unclear), yet in the medical field some medical professionals
have exploited these "gray areas" for their own financial
reason. They can easily take advantage of your fear and
anxiety to "coerce" you into unnecessary tests to generate
more income for themselves. Did you know that? Usually,
patients will not know it because they just received a very
"kind" treatment from the medical office. Worse than this is
a fraud in billing. For example, a billing is sent to you and/
or your insurance company for the test, or treatment, that
you never received. It is unfortunate, but such conditions
have existed and have been reported over the years. This is
why I would advise you to always examine and check the
medical billing you received. If there is any doubt in your
mind, do not hesitate to ask and verify it.

But, please do not get discouraged. There are excellent
and trustworthy medical professionals around that will give
you excellent care. For your peace of mind, I have set up a
list of questions for you to ask yourself in case you suspect
that your medical professional is not completely honest with
you, or if you believe that you are being taken advantage of.

Let us ask ourselves the following questions:

- *Do you believe that your doctor is ordering more tests and/or is treating you better than others because you have a good health insurance coverage?*

- *Do you believe that the kindness and generosity that is extended to you by a medical professional (when ordering tests and scheduling procedures) is obviously accomplished at the expense of someone else's money?*

- *Has your medical professional taken a thorough medical history and has given you a physical examination by him herself? And afterwards, did your doctor follow up with a logical explanation and plan that was considerate of your well being, time, and financial obligation?*

- *Does your medical professional frequently tell you that, "This is the best way," or "That is best for you," simply to attract and gain your trust and faith?*

- *Will the results of the tests change the way your medical professional will take care of you?*

An honest review of these five questions will enlighten you and help you understand what your medical professionals are really doing for you. Now, let us look into the details of these issues.

To begin with, for some medical professionals, making more money for better living and paying bills is a conflict of interest that tends to cloud their decision-making in the care of their patients. At such a juncture in life, honesty and integrity play a very important role in making a decision about how one should care for you and still avoid the pitfalls of such a conflict. As I said before, we fortunately still have many honest and capable medical professionals around. But watch out for the few that exercise their skills with a kind smile, a courteous attitude, and a good bedside manner to "mislead" and lure you into going along with more tests and procedures. They are very skillful and smooth at their deceptive ways. Under their seemingly "natural" expression of sympathy, kindness, generosity, and understanding, they've learned how to generate more – "personal income." And all of this is done because someone else, maybe you or your insurance companies, is willing to pay for everything.

Is there really anything best for you? Truthfully, there is no "one thing" best for you. At most, what medical professionals can say is, "This is something most reasonable for you," according to the available information at any given time. However (in the medical practice), patients frequently just want, and like, to hear what is best for them. But, there is no such a thing as "best for you". At most, "reasonable, or most reasonable, for you" is truly honest.

Are there too many tests for you? Let us ask ourselves, "If the test result will not change the treatment, why do the test?" Or, are the tests merely done for the sake of, "I would rather be safe than sorry," and "be safe" at the expense of someone else's money?

Knowing these odds in the medical practice will give you a cost-effective advantage of quality care. Meanwhile, if you have a good medical doctor, you will appreciate how lucky you are and what is being done for you.

Level 2: Drugs with Minimal Invasiveness

The introduction of sildenafil (Viagra, Pheizer, Inc.) in the middle of April, 1998 has changed the entire landscape of the sequence for administering medications for men's erectile difficulties.

Before then, I would have a patient once in a while who would tell me that someone, or a friend, has received some "special pills" or "an injection" that "this doctor" or "that doctor" gave them and restored their lost sex life. Usually, they have no idea what the name of the medications was. To them, there was some sense of a mystery or miracle. In fact, only five drugs are available for this level of care and have been used with some effectiveness to improve erection in some patients. Among these medications, sildenafil should be the first one to be mentioned for many reasons that will be discussed below.

a. Sildenafil (Viagra, Pfeizer, Inc.)

Sildenafil (Viagra) is the newest drug for treating erectile difficulties and has been available since mid-April, 1998. Its brand name, Viagra, will be used for discussion because of its high familiarity to general public. The Author has no financial connection with Pfeizer Inc.

Despite the price of $7.50 to $10 per tablet, Viagra has been the fastest sought, and prescribed, in drug history since its introduction because of its easy access and use, as well as its reasonable profile of safety.

There are three strengths of dosage, 25 mg, 50 mg, and 100 mg, to choose from. However, in general, it is most advisable to start out with the lowest dose, 25 mg; and slowly the dosage may be increased to meet the practical need. Unlike other medication, which needs to be used either right before intercourse (such as prostaglandin E1) or use on a regular basis (such as yohimbine and testosterone), it can be taken within 1 to three hours before sexual intercourse, although the onset of action can be as early as 30 to 60 minutes. In order to achieve an erection, a natural **mental** and **physical** sexual stimulation is still required. However, there is an absolute contraindication that is its use on the patients who are taking any forms of nitrates for coronary heart disease. The combined effect of blood vessel dilation from sildenafil (Viagra) and nitrates can produce a dramatic drop in blood pressure, which may precipitate a fatal heart attack or stroke. Other side effects are headaches (15%), flushing (10%), indigestion (7%), nasal congestion (5%), and temporary change in color or brightness of vision (2-3%). Unlike papaverine, phentolamine, or alprostdil, there has been no report of the occurrence of priapism (unwanted prolonged erection).

Conversely, if a man took sildenafil (Viagra) for sexual intercourse and developed a heart attack, he should not use any nitrate (such as nitroglycerine) for self-relief, and should inform his medical provider of his special clinical situation of having used Viagra for intercourse and developed a subsequent heart attack. Why? Again, the combined use of sildenafil and nitrate can induce a severe drop of blood pressure and make the clinical condition worse. So, be careful!

How does Viagra work on the penis to produce an erection? Under normal mental and physical sexual stimulation, a substance, *nitric oxide* (NO), will be released from the sponge bodies of the penis. NO then activates an enzyme, *guanylate cyclase*, to produce a substance called *cyclic guanosine monophosphate* (cGMP). This cGMP is the real substance to relax the smooth muscles inside the sponge bodies, so a natural erection takes place. After orgasm and ejaculation, the supply of nitric oxide (NO) is turned off, the existing amount of cGMP is then degraded timely through the help of an enzyme, PDE type 5. And penile erection gradually subsides and disappears.

Sildanifil (Viagra) has the effect to block the enzyme, PDE type 5, to degrade cGMP. Subsequently, the amount of cGMP inside the sponge bodies increases and its effect to relax the smooth muscles of sponge bodies is greatly enhanced. In other words, it simply enhances the natural process of an erection.

As for any drug, it is not a panacea. If the circulation and nerve supply to the penis is so impaired, the effect of Viagra will still not be sufficient to generate a satisfactory erection for sexual intercourse. Furthermore, due to its ultimate clinical effect to help patients recover their lost pleasure from sexual intercourse and its easy availability to cover the expense, some patients tend to pump up their mental expectation and overlook their physical fitness to act and the contraindication of the drug. As a result, its overuse, and even abuse, are likely. Therefore some undue harms to personal health, especially for those patients of coronary heart disease (with or without using nitrates) may occur. The worst of them may be a fatal heart attack.

As is well known to us, emotional and/or physical over-exertion may lead to a heart attack, and even death, in the patients with coronary heart disease! As previously stated, sexual intercourse is a life experience of a heavy mental and physical drainage. Therefore, it is easy to imagine how many men could, and would, die of heart attack that is precipitated by overexertion during sexual intercourse. However, for the sake of "social grace", only a heart attack is mentioned as the cause of death although sexual intercourse is indeed the real, initial responsibility. Therefore, it is mandatory to know, and appreciate, Nature and the goals of sex life as described in Parts I and III before using Viagra for your "real" benefit.

In short, please remember; truly enjoy sex, but don't allow the pursuit and enjoyment of sex to cause undue expectation and/or over-exertion. Instead, be sure to use Viagra wisely and judiciously to really enhance the quality of life for you and your partner. For individual details of care, sex counseling, and the use of Viagra, please check with your own personal physician.

b. Phentoloamine:

This drug can block the ability of sympathetic nerves to contract the smooth muscles of vessels. Thereby, it then relaxes the smooth muscles of vessels so that blood vessels dilate, blood to the penis increases, and an erection develops. Its effect of dilating blood vessels at the dose of 40 mg of oral use may take place within 20 to 30 minutes. Its side effects are nasal stuffiness and flushing. Its effectiveness was described as moderate. It is worthwhile to try and see.

c. Apomorphine:

This drug should be taken by placing it beneath the tongue at a dose of 2 mg. Its action starts inside the brain (central) by blocking the effect of dopamine. As a result, like phentolamine by mouth, it can induce penile erection in some patients within 20 to 30 minutes after use. As with any drug, it may have some side effects such as slight nausea (5-10%) at a low dose of 2 mg, and even rare, fainting spell at a high dose of 5-6 mg.

d. Yohimbine:

Over the last four decades, yohimbine has been off and on the market for its use to enhance erections. Yohimbine is mainly extracted from a plant, *corynanthe yohimbe,* although it is also found in various plants. The real mechanism for its effectiveness in improving erections is not yet completely understood. However, the available information suggests that the effects possibly responsible for improving erections is that Yohimbine is a central nerve stimulant and causes the smooth muscles inside the penis to relax.

It is given by mouth at a dose of 5.4 mg three times a day. Its use is usually safe. Occasionally, there are side effects such as headache, not sleeping well, shivering, etc. After Viagra, its use has dramatically decreased. However, it is still useful for some patients because of its low costs.

e. Testosterone:

It can be given by month (oral), or through muscle (intra-muscular) injection, or even by a patch on the skin (transdermal, such as *Androderm* from SmithKline Beecham Pharmaceuticals). Intramuscular injection is preferable because of its reliable absorption to provide a good testosterone blood level. Both the routes through mouth and skin are useful because of their noninvasive nature. **But the real need for testosterone is not common and is required far less than patients and most medical professionals would believe.** In general, if you have a good sexual desire and a good physical appearance of manhood, it is very unlikely for you to have a deficiency of testosterone and you rarely need it. Because of this fact, it is advisable to test the testosterone blood level with a proper interpretation before its use. To follow the effect of using testosterone, a repeated blood test for testosterone level may be required. In addition, a test for liver function is needed due to the fact that some damage to the liver in certain patients may result from the long-term use of testosterone. Of caution, it should never be used for patients having prostate cancer because testosterone can accelerate the growth of prostate cancer.

The side effects from using a drug are the common anxiety and concern of many patients. However, in reality, it is impossible for any medical professional to predict which side effects may happen to you. The only sure way to know if you will have certain side effects from a drug or not is your personal repetitive use of the medication. Therefore, it is important to cooperate with your medical professionals to watch for the possible occurrence of any side effects. Generally, it would be more practical for you to simply use the recommended drug and observe your response. But definitely keep in touch with your medical professional who gave you the prescription if any suspicion of side effects arises.

Usually, testosterone is used only on a trial basis for about one month. If it is helpful in improving your erection, it is reasonable to continue its use. If not, it is advisable to test the blood level of testosterone. If the testosterone level is normal, its use is then discontinued. But please do not get disappointed. For further steps of care of your erectile difficulties, your medical professional will guide you through step by step.

Despite having various drugs to choose from, there are still more drugs under investigation for their clinical trial and use for improving erection, such as vasoactive intestinal polypeptide (VIP), a potent smooth muscle relaxant. As expected, even more of its kind will surely emerge because no single drug would be perfect and effective for all. Nonetheless, medical technology has made many solid strides in developing the drugs for erectile difficulties over the last two decades.

Level 3: Assisted erection

If you failed to respond to the care from Levels 0, 1, and 2, now it is the time to move along to the care of Level 3. The treatment options at this level are more invasive and expensive. Their use will give patients an immediate physical discomfort or pain although an instant result in a good erection may be expected for many patients. Because of the nature of their usage, both patients and sexual partners would require more intense mental counseling and adjustment to diffuse their potential mental barrier in order to accept these treatment options for their active sexual rehabilitation. Three options are available for this level of care.

Option a. Injectable or Insertable Drug(s):

Three injectable drugs have been used for the purpose of achieving an erection. They are papaverine, phentolamine (Regitine), and prostaglandin E1 (alprostadil) and can be used alone or in combination. However, only Prostaglandin E1 (alprostadil) is approved by the Food Drug Administration (FDA). All three drugs are given usually by self-injection into the spongy bodies at the locations of 2 or 10 o'clock at the back part of the penis, (Figure 4). The mechanism for these drugs to work and initiate an erection relies on their ability to relax the smooth muscles inside the sponge bodies of the penis from their direct contact with them. As a result, the blood flow to the penis increases, blood is then entrapped and accumulated inside the sponge bodies to block the venous blood flow out of the penis, and an erection develops.

There are two brands of self-injectable alprostadil. They are called *Caverject*, Pharmacia & Upjohn, or *Edex*, Schwarz Pharma, Inc. However, among these three drugs, alprostadil is the only one that can be given through the urethra (channel) with the form of suppository under a brand name, MUSE, Vivus, Inc., which will be discussed on page 159 under **Option b**.

The injectable alprostadil has been observed to have a positive response rate of about 75%. However, maybe due to the price, and the invasive nature of an injection, a high discontinuation rate has been noted in most clinical studies. As with any drug, self penile injection of these drugs may have the following side effects such as prolonged erection (priapism) at <1%, pain at 10-20%, and scar tissue formation from chronic use. If the scar formation is severe, the penis will curve at erection just like the condition of Peyronie's disease. In addition, the injectable alprostadil has its own

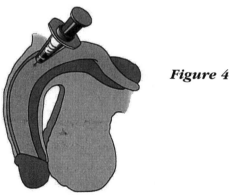

Figure 4

Intracavernosal Injection

contraindications, hence, it is not recommended to be used in men with a history of hypersensitivity to the drug, at risk for developing priapism (sickle cell disease or other hyper-coagulable conditions), taking monoamine oxidase inhibitors.

For more details of dosages and possible complications of these drugs, please check with your own medical professional or the PDR (Physician Desk Reference). One of the notable complications that you should know is prolonged erection (priapism). In general, it is not advisable to let the drug-induced erection last longer than three (3) hours. If it does happen, you should have emergency care to reverse the unwanted, severe, prolonged erection. This is usually achieved with a medication to contract the smooth muscles of the sponge bodies inside the penis. For more details of the clinical implication of this occurrence, please check with your own medical professional.

In general, without proper instruction, practice, and supervision from a competent medical professional, you are not advised to administer these drugs by yourself. This precaution is for your own safety. To illustrate the importance of this precaution, I would like to present to you my personal experience in three unfortunate patients as follows:

Case 1: *I had a physician as a patient that happened to be a retired urologist. His impotence occurred after his total prostate removal for prostate cancer. His radical prostate surgery has controlled his cancerous disease very well for more than 10 years. For his erectile difficulty, he confirmed using papaverine through self-penile injection, which he saw on a television show. I then explained to him the current thoughts of using* *that drug by self-injection. I also urged him to see me first. However, for whatever his reasons were, he did not. And he was quite confident and gave himself the injection of papaverine. After the facts of self-penile injection and the occurrence of priapism, the history of his unfortunate events was obtained. It was noted that after the first injection, he achieved only a partial erection, which was not rigid enough for vaginal penetration in his attempt to have sexual intercourse. He then gave himself a second dose of papaverine of injection to his penis. The second injection indeed induced a rigid erection, enough for intercourse, but it lasted much longer than what he needed. Unfortunately, he did not seek emergency care to reverse the unwanted prolonged erection, which lasted more than 12 hours. Eventually, he went to the emergency room of a local hospital where he was treated. After this incidence, he was no longer able to have an erection, even through self-injection with papaverine. Later, I performed an implantation of an inflatable penile prosthesis for him as the final resort of sexual rehabilitation. So far, he has been doing well with it.*

Case 2: *The patient was a 55 years old retired physician who saw me only sporadically for his slow urine flow. For his poor erection, he kept this concern to himself. After his own search, he gave himself an injection of Prostaglandin E1 to his penis. Only a poor erection was observed after the injection. Unfortunately, he developed the extensive sloughing (necrosis) of the skin of his penis after the self injection of Prostaglandin E1 to his penis. It took more than five months to heal. In reviewing the sequence of the unfortunate events, it* *was noted that he probably did not inject correctly into the inside of the sponge bodies of the penis, but instead injected to the outside of it. Afterwards, he was found to have low blood testosterone. Fortunately, his ability to have an erection was restored by giving him a supplement of testosterone.*

Case 3: *The patient was a 46-years old gentleman, an autoworker. He came to see me with his wife for his inability in intercourse because of poor erection. Through his medical history, it was noted that he had suffered from a severe stroke that left him with one-half of his body not able to move easily, called hemiparesis. Due to his disability, and its subsequent side effects after the severe stroke, the relationship of this couple almost went down the drain. They were very upset and angry with one another in spite of their verbal denial concerning the significance of patient's inability to achieve an erection (which was the cause of their current marital discord). And through my usual approach, as previously described, I was able to bring this couple to face, and recognize, the truth of the issues. It took me more than four months to slowly rehabilitate his sexual difficulties. But finally, we settled down to a treatment option with penile injection of Prostaglandin E1 by his wife because of his manual disability from the severe stroke. Currently, they are still together, are well and reasonably happy with their sexual relationship.*

The first two disappointing examples were not used to scare you. Instead, they were used as advice for you to work closely with your own medical professional, even though you may have your own idea of good care. As long as you use common sense, are properly instructed, and co-operate with your own well-experienced medical professional, the odds that you may have such misfortunes are almost impossible. Even if a mishap, such as a severely prolonged erection, does happen, it can be timely reversed. And the late, adverse effects from a prolonged erection can be minimized, or even avoided.

The third example is used to demonstrate what the variations and complexities that might be confronted in the process of evaluation and care for male erectile difficulties, and what is required before a successful sexual rehabilitation can be achieved. Therefore, please be confident in what a medical professional can do for you. The key to success in this particular field is knowledge, understanding, and team-work.

Option b. Intraurethral Suppository of Alprostadil:

As stated in *Option a*, alprostadil (prostaglandin E1) is the only drug that can be given through the urethra (channel) with a suppository, (Figure 5), it is manufactured by Vivus, Inc. under the brand name of *MUSE*. The dose of alprostadil (about 125 to 1,000 micrograms) is much higher than that (5 to 40 micrograms) used in its injectable form, Caverject or Edex. About 50% of men receiving a suppository of alprostadil at home can achieve successful intercourse.

Before inserting a suppository of alprostadil into the urethra, please be sure that you have read and understand the details of technical instructions of insertion in order to minimize local injury to the urethra. As of any drug, MUSE has its following side effects in a decreasing order. They may include local ache in the penis, legs, and in the area behind

Figure 5

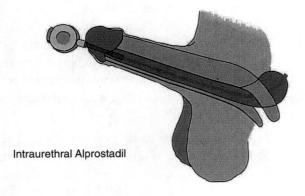

Intraurethral Alprostadil

the scrotum (sac), warming or burning sensation in the urethra, redness of the penis, minor bleeding or spotting from the urethra, prolonged erection (priapism), swelling of leg veins, low blood pressure (3 to 4%), light-headedness or dizziness, fainting spells (0.4%), and rapid pulse. In spite of these side effects, the use of alprostadil through the urethra is relatively safe and moderately effective in managing erectile difficulties. For further details, and before using this treatment option, please check and clarify your questions with your medical professionals.

Option c: Vacuum Constriction Devices (VCD):

Vacuum Constriction Devices (VCD) illustrated in Figure 6 on the following page; the name itself explicitly describes its mechanism of producing an erection. As you can see from the illustration on the following page, this device consists of a long cylinder and a pump, which can be operated

Figure 6

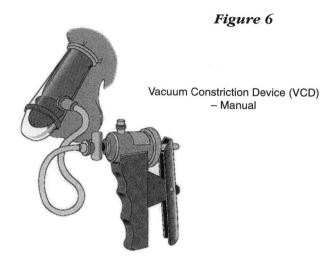

Vacuum Constriction Device (VCD)
– Manual

manually or electrically. The cylinder is applied onto the pendulous (hanging) part of the penis with a seal around its base. The pump is then operated to suck the air out of the cylinder to produce a negative pressure. This resulting negative pressure draws blood to fill up the penis and produce an erection. Meanwhile, a well-designed elastic constriction band is then placed around the base of the penis to prevent the blood already inside the penis from escaping. As a result, a satisfactory erection can be achieved and maintained for completing sexual intercourse.

VCD is a well-established, non-invasive treatment option and has been approved by the Food and Drug Administration (FDA) for over-the-counter purchase. However, it is still most advisable to use it under the instructions and supervision of the experienced, medical professionals. Due to the physical appearance of VCD, potential inconvenience, and request for manual skills, an adequate counseling to promote the mental acceptance of VCD is needed before its use. And both the patient and/or their sexual partner may use a VCD comfortably.

Because of the mechanical nature of VCD, the patients may experience penile discomfort, pain, numbness, bruising, and retarded ejaculation. To minimize these potential adverse effects, proper skill of using VCD is required and a limit in usage time of 30 minutes is advised. Despite these adverse effects, VCD has been effective to rehabilitate sexual function for about 80 - 90% of men with erectile difficulties.

Many forms of VCD are designed, and available, from many companies such as Mission Pharmacal Company, NuMedtec Inc., Osbon Medical Systems, etc. But each one serves the same purpose of use. Its price varies from $300 to $500. In general, its purchase price may be lower if it is acquired directly from a medical office because of the promotion of manufacturer's professional discount to physicians.

To ease the burden of redundancy and inconvenience, let us compare the carrying, exercise, and use of VCD for the enjoyment of sexual intercourse to those of golf clubs and bag for the recreational enjoyment of golfing. For preparing themselves to go on a golf field and enjoy the joy of golfing, golfers are willing to spend a big sum of money to purchase clubs, carrying bag, walking shoes, golf balls, gloves, and so on. In addition, they are further willing to pay golf instructors to teach them how to play golf correctly. After the instructive course, they will also take time to practice how to position themselves in order to swing the clubs and hit golf balls correctly and efficiently. In other words, they make every effort by dedicating their time and attention to improve their golfing for the purpose of having fun from golfing.

How about using VCD for sexual enjoyment? A similar scenario in preparation, effort, and practice of using VCD should be applied for your sexual rehabilitation. Does this make sense to you? To reach the goal of medical care, we all need to pay a certain price for it. This reality should be understandable to anyone. With this scene in mind, you will be more willing to try the use of VCD.

Level 4: Implantation of Penile Prosthesis

This level of care is considered as the last resort for active sexual rehabilitation. Penile implant has been proven to be effective and safe for the last three decades. Before the increasing availability of the methods for assisted erection with vacuum constriction device (VCD), direct application of Prostaglandin E1, Papaverine, and Phentoloamine in 1990's, and the newest addition of Sildanifil (Viagra), it was the most popular means for active sexual rehabilitation back in 1970's and 1980's.

The implantation of a penile prosthesis is the most invasive among all the means of care for active sexual rehabilitation. Because of its invasive nature, I would like to give some details about the choices of penile prosthesis, the surgical procedure, and the clinical implication of its practical use. For further individual details, please, always check with your own medical professional.

When Would You Need an Implantation of Penile Prosthesis?

As repeatedly stated, it is considered to be the last resort for active sexual rehabilitation of erectile dysfunction. After a patient fails to respond to all the available conservative treatment options, an implantation of penile prosthesis may be considered as the most reasonable means of active sexual rehabilitation.

A decision to implant a penile prosthesis can be reached through an honest and thorough assessment, and under the consideration and cooperation of the patient, the sexual partner, and the urologist. But, please remember; you, the patient, are the one who makes the final decision.

Why is it Better to Have a Joint Decision?

However, while a man legally has his right to make a final decision for the fate of his body, a joint decision is still most reasonable, and desirable, for the matter of sexual inter-

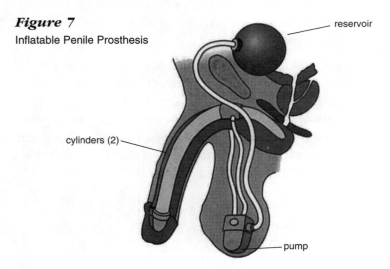

***Figure* 7**
Inflatable Penile Prosthesis

reservoir

cylinders (2)

pump

course because of the obvious involvement of two parties.

In addition, it is because a joint effort will take the well-being of both parties into consideration. Such a final decision should most truly represent the practical need rather than simply what the patient wants or desires.

How Many Kinds of Penile Prosthesis are Available?

Based on the degree of cost and complexity of its components and operation, there are three types of penile prosthesis to choose from. They are **malleable penile prosthesis, self-contained penile prosthesis,** and (illustrated below) **inflatable penile prosthesis**. Among these three, the malleable one is simplest in structure and least costly. The inflatable penile prosthesis is most complicated and costly. But it is still quite easy to use after the patient (with a good manual dexterity) is properly instructed. The self-contained prosthesis lies somewhere in between the other two. The malleable one is easiest to use and the inflatable one requires the highest level of manual dexterity to operate. And again, the self-contained one is in between. Technically, it is not difficult to use them as long as the mind is clear and the patient has a reasonable manual skill. However, if a patient's memory and manual skills are impaired, the malleable one would be the most reasonable choice.

For an easier understanding, please allow me to draw an analogy. It would be appropriate to use a car for transportation as an analogy to compare penile prosthesis for sexual intercourse. A person will purchase a car for "personal reasons" and at different prices, depending upon what kind of car and price a person is willing to pay. To understand and imagine what a person would purchase in a penile prosthesis; a malleable penile prosthesis is just like owning a Ford

Escort, a self-contained prosthesis is like owning a Ford Taurus, and an inflatable prosthesis is like owning a Ford Lincoln Continental. In other words, a person will get what they pay for, although they are all used for the same basic reason.

How Does a Penile Prosthesis Work for You?

As was explained in Part II, the penis is composed of three cylinder-like structures, including a **single ventral tube (corpus spongiosum)** mainly used for urine to pass through, and the **two paired tubes (corpora cavernosa)** in its dorsal, mainly responsible for an erection. The mid-cross section may look like the "funny face" of a clown. The penile prosthesis is basically paired cylinder structures which may be surgically placed snugly inside the dorsal paired cylinders, or the corpora cavernosa of the penis. And a well-positioned penile prosthesis will allow a man to have an instant "artificial" erection **whenever a man's optimal readiness of mental comfort to perform and the physical fitness to act is reasonable and available.** Although a penile prosthesis can generate an instant erection, it would not be to the best interest of a man if he is not mentally and physically ready to have intercourse. As everyone knows, a full course of sexual activities is very mentally and physically draining, and sexual fantasies may lead to overuse and indulgence. This situation could be harmful to the general health and welfare of the patient after all.

What are the General Surgical Aspects of Implanting a Penile Prosthesis?

The actual surgery to implant a penile prosthesis is usually done under spinal, or general, anesthesia and under a very

strict aseptic environment. A high level of skill in surgery
and aseptic techniques of a urological surgeon and team
will usually provide an excellent result with a very low rate
of complications, such as infection, perforation of the sheaths
of spongy bodies, buckling (crooked) prosthesis, etc. The
sites of incision are usually around the base of the penis, at
either the front or back side. The surgical time is usually
about one to two and one-half hours, depending upon the
type of prosthesis implanted and the skills and experience
of the surgeon. The length of the hospital stay is about zero
to two days. Further detailed information of an individual's
care should be directed towards an experienced surgeon
and his/her team.

How Can You Overcome the Possible Fear of Surgery for the Implantation of a Penile Prosthesis?

As a general understanding, invasive surgery is the last
alternative of care that will provide a result of care that "conservative means" could not achieve. Of course, surgery always carries some risks of complications. Notably for penile
prosthesis, the commonly mentioned complications that may
arise are infection and perforation of penile tube-like structures. Fortunately, these mishaps are very rare if the surgery
is done under an environment of strict aseptic techniques
by a well-trained, experienced, and skillful urological surgeon and team.

However, very occasionally, there may be a patient who
demands a result of absolutely no side effects or complications from surgery or medical care. He/she is looking for the
best of the best. That, of course, is an excellent quest for
life. But in the reality of life, it is impossible. Common sense
has told, and taught, us the universal rule of cause and ef-

fect. **Therefore, the only way to absolutely avoid any potential complications or side effects is to do nothing because there is nothing, or no one, to be blamed.**

To further this understanding, I share a "real but sarcastic" joke with an occasional patient by saying, "Mr. So and So, if you insist on having a perfect result and absolutely having no complication, I really cannot do it for you. However, there are two 'persons' who you may go and consult." Such a patient will brighten his/her eyes and eagerly says, "Oh! Who are they?" I calmly reply in a smile, "Do you really want to know?" The patient will be eager to insist and answer, "Yes, of course, I would." Then I respond and say, "Well, these two persons I just mentioned are the ones who have no privileges to take care of you directly in the real life. The first one is God. To have the help from God, you would need to pray. But God never tells you anything directly. The second one is a lawyer. Why? Because a lawyer would be by one-quarter inch better than any doctor at the time they sue a doctor for medical malpractice, even though most times a lawyer did never go to a medical school or have any real medical training. And a lawyer also has no obligation to take care of you." At this end, usually, the patient was well amused, and said with a smile, "I understand and agree. You are right." He/she clearly, and quickly, returned to a realistic world of life.

Again, as stated before, **medical professionals are doing their jobs to make your body and mind to work for you only as well, and as long, as possible. That is all they can, and will, do for you.**

To further ease the fear of surgery, please allow me to use an example of a patient going to have surgery for a hip replacement (due to severe degenerative hip joint disease):

The surgery for hip replacement, although a common surgery today, should not be undertaken lightly. But before the surgery takes place, almost every patient would go through a course of conservative care. This disease causes irritation from inflammation in and around the hip joint. At the very beginning of the disease, a patient may just feel some mild to moderate pain. A medical professional may simply prescribe a non-steroid, anti-inflammatory medication to decrease inflammation and ease pain. This basic conservative measure will help many patients for a good period of time. However, as the disease advances, medication alone will not sufficiently ease the pain or discomfort, and keep patients well in their walking function. Therefore, a high level of care will be reasonably required. Usually, you would need to have a combination of medication, such as some injections into the hip joints, and systemic physical therapy to maintain an active and passive range of motion in the hip joints with the use of a cane or a walker. This level of care may prove to be effective enough for some patients for a period of time. Eventually, some of the patients will need to have further care in order to maintain their mobility, such as total hip replacement surgery (artificial hip joint). Unfortunately, these patients may require such a surgery as the last resort for hip joint rehabilitation.

A similar scenario of progressive care for male erectile difficulties, applicable for sexual rehabilitation, is described in Section 19, from level 0 to level 4. And level 4 with penile implantation is the last resort of care.

At the time of deciding if a patient needs a penile implant, the patient would need to honestly ask himself if he would have good use of a penile implantation. Of course, it is always very important to be sure that your mental and physical readiness can be afforded without harming your general health or well-being. Otherwise, the penile implant, under negative circumstances, would not be worthwhile. I am not discouraging anyone from having this procedure for an active sexual rehabilitation. Instead, I just want to again remind everyone from my heart, to be sure if the penile implant is really needed. I hope this comparison will help people make a wise and reasonable decision about their future medical and health needs.

In my practice as a urologist, I have had patients that pleaded with me to have the penile prosthesis. Even though their mental and physical states were not ready, they wanted a penile implant so badly that they would've done, or paid, anything for the operation. And after a period of intense counseling, they changed their minds about the operation. This point of "surgery necessity" verses "surgery desire" is clearly seen between the patient needing a total hip replacement and a patient desiring a penile implant.

It has been a proven fact that a long-term immobilization of patients who suffer from a disabled hip/joint disease (caused by degenerative joint disease or hip fracture) will lead to an early death. In other words, without a hip replacement, the patients with disabled hip/joint diseases would die earlier because of immobilization and the related complications. But a patient that does not receive a penile implant will most likely live as long as the one with a penile prosthesis because he has no concern of mortality from immobilization and other complications.

Through an understanding of what we have discussed so far, I deeply believe anyone would be able to make a very sound decision as to what level of care is really needed, and not just what the patient wants, or what medical professionals promise they can do. Now, if there comes a time in one's life that that the highest level of sexual intimacy (intercourse) is not in the best interest of a person's overall health, please understand that the contents of a sex life can be reasonably fulfilling, rewarding, and satisfactory without intercourse. Survival is essential for life and should come first. I hope that most of my readers would agree with this "point of view", although occasionally someone might emotionally be charged and say, "I would rather have a moment of fun with intercourse than live without it." But ultimately, the decision is "yours".

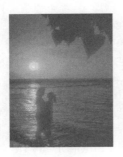

While the real value of a traditional wisdom indeed exists, at times, it could be very difficult to prove or disprove it in scientific research. At such a juncture, and to benefit from it, the use of common sense and moderation is the rescue for this uncertainty.

20

A Few Words on Nutrition, Herbs, "Accessories", and Sex

Without a mention of nutrition, herbs, and "accessories" for sex life, the task of this book seems far from its completness because some discussions on these items have been the common topics in many publications. Too many laypersons are curious and commonly ask questions about these products. While I am not an expert in these areas, I am still obligated to express my views on these subjects for your consideration and reference.

In everyone's life, it has become common sense that good nutrition, good exercise, and a good mind-set are essential for a good performance of any task; it is of no exception to sex life as discussed before.

To have a good nutritional status, a "balanced" diet with all edibles around Nature is the sure way to reach this goal.

However, the luxury of having a balanced diet has been disturbed and distorted, if not destroyed, by changing natural habitats, commercialism, and subsequent changes in lifestyles. As a result, many individuals may suffer from chronic malnutrition with a shortage of certain vitamins or minerals although they still look healthy. On the other hand, many commercial companies are taking advantage of this nutritional concern and fear to promote the consumption of multiple vitamins, mineral supplements, and others to enhance vigor and even longevity. Such conflicting messages may catch you in between. However, there is no excellent solution to it. It is reasonable to use your common sense and a middle stance in taking nutritional supplements in moderation, not under obsession.

In general, a balanced intake of proteins, fats, and carbohydrates with a touch of supplement of multivitamins and minerals is reasonably advisable. This approach to diet will keep you nutritionally in reasonably good shape and its information is readily available from most medical offices or elsewhere. But be sure to avoid becoming overweight if possible.

The foods containing essential metabolite phosphorus, calcium, magnesium, and zinc have been suggested and reported to improve sexual drive and responsiveness. Among them, phosphorus has been the most sharply focused. In many instances, a solid convincing evidence is still lacking. Therefore, if you choose to use them, just use them in moderation and see what happens to you. Does a supplement do you any good? Fairly speaking, your personal repetitive experience could tell you the "real" story, no one else can, especially while there is no clear evidence to support its use from today's scientific research. But please remember the facts that many of the supplements are natural products and have been used for thousands of years by many cultures and races. Yet the claims of their beneficial effects continue to spread. For instance, Brewer's yeast, wheat bran, pumpkin seeds, squash seeds, wheat germ, sunflower seeds, etc. are found to have a high content of phosphorus; kelp, Swiss cheese, chedder cheese, etc., for calcium; kelp, wheat bran, wheat germ, almonds, cashews, etc., for magnesium; fresh oysters, ginger root, black pepper, etc., for zinc.

As for herbs, some 40,000 of 800,000 species of plants on the Earth have been studied. But only 20% of these were found useful for health enhancement. The commonly mentioned examples for sexual enhancement have been ginseng, spirulina, honeybee pollen, royal jelly, honey, damiana, yohimbe, etc. They are natural foods. Much of their sexual enhancing effects are believed to result from their high contents of certain nutritions such as vitamins A, B-complex, C, E, zinc, phosphorus, etc., or their direct or indirect effects on the muscles of the penis. Again, if you are inspired and want to use them, be sure to do some your own home work about the natures of these natural supplements or consult your medical professionals before you use them in moderation, with care and no obsession.

Understandably, an increase in the supply of needed nutritions in the case of shortage may improve the bodily functions, including sexual function. Please remember that a constant use of any supplement can exert an effect of selfawareness to promote some placebo effect as well. At times, you may wonder if the supplement that you are taking is really helpful for you. At such a juncture of wandering, again, let your body's repetitive experience to tell the "real" story of its effectiveness.

How about "accessories" for sex life? Various perfumes for men and women have been used to simulate the scent effect of natural pheromones such as female copulins in the vaginal fluid. As well, many varieties of different clothes and dresses, mainly for women, have been designed to enhance sexual arousal by exaggerating visual intimate effects. As a result, a person's mind is sexually enticed. Which one may work well for you? Who knows? Again, your personal experience with common sense will prove to you one way or the other. You would need to explore yourself. Again, do not overuse it with obsession.

I hope the above information and view can serve as your reference to decide for your own sexual adventure.

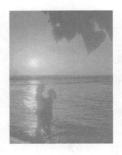

A periodic genuine and cooperative review of the effectiveness of treatment with medical professionals will maximize the benefit of care.

21

Reassessment of the Effects of Treatment

No matter what kind of treatment you have received, it is mandatory to have a series of follow-up visits with your medical professionals on a reasonable schedule to review the plus or minus of the outcome of care for erectile difficulties. During a visit, an evaluation of objective, and subjective, improvement (or deterioration) can be done and recorded. Your further questions about your medical care can be answered as your medical professional can fine-tune your care with such necessary adjustments as the dosage of a drug and the techniques of operating a device that can be adjusted and corrected, if necessary. At the end, your medical professionals want to be sure that the care you are receiving is compatible with your physical and psychosocial needs, and general health.

In case the result of care is not as good as you may expect, please do not make your own decision to discontinue the method of care as originally agreed, or refuse to make a return visit to your medical professional, and complain and get upset. It would be in the best interest of all parties to jointly review the details of the past and present care in order to map out a reasonable solution to your concern or dissatisfaction. Please remember, medical professionals are humans as you are; they will do the most reasonable things for you according to their training and experience.

Case Study: *RL, a 65 year old healthy man came to see me for a persistent recurrence of spontaneous erection of his inflatable penile prosthesis for three months. History revealed he underwent a procedure to implant his currently malfunctioning prothesis in Florida a year earlier. Then a persistent recurrence of spontaneous erection developed and he suffered pain and embarrassment from it. Through a careful evaluation, it is noted that the problem was from the malfunction of the pump device of penile prosthesis. Nonetheless, some manual efforts to reverse the condition was provided but failed. After a lengthy discussion, we agreed to replace the whole system of inflatable penile prosthesis . This second surgery resolved his problem for three months. However, later he seemed noting he was not able to deflate the prosthesis as before. Then he returned to my clinic where he was given more instructions on operating the pump device after listening to his concern and identifying the problem. Since then, he has been able to operate his penile prothesis well.*

This case is to illustrate the need for a close follow-up with your medical professional timely and cooperatively. While nothing in medical care is perfect, most medical problems could be managed and solved in a reasonable and sensible way.

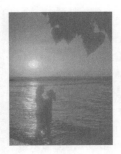

Largely speaking, greed and no real cash coming out of one's own pocket (medical professionals and patients alike) have led to overuse and abuse.

22

A Few Words of Caution of Overuse, and Abuse of Devices or Medications for Erection

As explored and defined in prior discussion, sex life can be viewed as a gift from God for humans to enhance the bonds of society by improving their quality of life. Meanwhile, it is clearly realized that the full course of life is an experience of a heavy mental and physical drainage.

Many a man has a high expectation to enjoy more pleasure from more sexual intercourse and ejaculation. However, there are times when his mental condition is not ready to perform and his physical ability is not sufficient to act. Then it is not wise to force himself to initiate erection, intercourse, orgasm, and ejaculation.

However, if he does it anyway under negative mental and/ or physical conditions, the result of his sexual acts will not enhance the quality of life for him and his sexual partner. Instead, it will harm him and the relationship. Worst, it may claim his life. Therefore, I strongly recommend a man to cautiously remind himself of using common sense and honestly listening to what his body signals to him. With such a precaution in mind, an overuse or abuse will be easily minimized and avoided.

Furthermore, financially, it could be a social and ethical issue. While most people have a good insurance coverage for medical care, the bottom line is the cost incurred. Who will pay for it? Directly, employers pay; however, indirectly, we all pay for it. For the sake of social conscience and reality of cost-effectiveness, we all should respect and observe a high moral standard that **we should not accomplish our deeds of kindness and generosity at the expense of someone else's money, as many politicians, attorneys, and other professionals do every day**. Under many circumstances, and in some sense, what they are operating is, more or less, like a form of licensed robbery, even like a form of Mafia as a group. The fact is that it is nothing illegal, but very unethical. The common feature of their behaviors is to serve their self-interest under a hidden (invisible) coverage of providing a quality service and the best interest of people but, in the very truth, all at the expense of someone else's money and suffering. Unfortunately, most of the people can not recognize it because of the reasons as mentioned before, or are even afraid to reveal it. At our current peaking time of increasing complicity of the laws and the fight for control and self-interest, it would be beneficial for all of us to remind ourselves of this reality of a society.

At times, I saw patients with a health insurance from which he/she will not need to pay a penny for any medical care under the policy. These patients tend to be very demanding and frequently say, "Dr. Lin, I would rather be safe than sorry. Please do anything you could to help me," even after a lengthy and careful process of history taking, physical examination, discussion, and explanation.

Usually, they look and act so kindly and generously that they would draw due respect from anyone. On some occasions, I told such patients that, "I know you are very anxious. But according to my training, experience, and all the works I just did for you, there is no need to do further tests. But we need to work together under a close observation and I will see you in a couple of weeks." However, some might still insist to have more tests, and even surgery. Under such a circumstance, at times, I asked, "If you would need to pay about 25% of the incurred cost with the cash from your own pocket, would you want them?" In my experience, there has been almost no exception that the patient would smile, shake head, and say, "No." An almost identical conversation has been experienced with some medical professionals under a similar scenario. Unfortunately, the "funny" money of insurance or public resources and humans' greedy nature tend to deceive the mind and conscience of many people.

Again, luckily we do have many honest and capable medical professionals. If not, we would never have our current landscape of medical care and advancement for us to receive. However, with the described scenes in mind, we all together can do much better for our society and next generation to come.

To the very truth, a desire for the selfishness due to whatever the value is, is the most real initiative of an act.

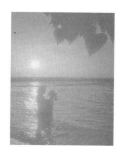

Disorders of Desire (libido) 23

As discussed extensively in prior sections, a satisfactory combination of a man's mental comfort to perform and physical fitness to act is essential for a man's successful sexual performance. With no, or impaired, desire to initiate sexual behaviors, it is impossible to unfold a full scene of romantic sexual acts for anyone.

If a man is experiencing a decrease in his sexual desire, it is useful for him to honestly examine and answer the following questions:

- *Does the loss of sexual desire come to me slowly over a period of time, or suddenly after a special event? If it occurred slowly, how long has it been and how did it progress? If suddenly, did it happen after any special event? And did it progress persistently or intermittently?*

- *Did you recently have any unusual stress resulting from the events that are related with your interpersonal relationship with sexual partner, financial burden, professional or job security, or family dispute over any important issues such as social, personal, ideological, or even political issues, etc.?*

- *Are you experiencing a major physical insult from a disease and/or its related treatment? A man receiving medical chemotherapy for a cancerous disease is a common example.*

After reviewing and answering a series of specific questions, you will be examined by your medical professional. Usually your medical professional would like to focus on looking for any signs of potential hormonal disorders such as testicular atrophy, a change of vision, unusual hair or fat distribution of the body, etc. After these efforts, a general impression as to the causes for your loss of desire may be suspected. Then he/she may order some tests to verify the suspicion of hormonal disorders. Fortunately, the hormonal disorders as the cause for the loss of sexual desire are rare.

If the loss of desire is persistent, the underlying reason for it may be physical, such as the above mentioned hormonal disorders. If it has been off and on, some psychogenic factors may be blamed. Commonly, it is depression leading to performance anxiety, or fear usually due to a situational change of time, location, or partner.

With the background of the knowledge as briefly mentioned, it should be helpful for you to initiate some thoughts and practice of self-help or correction. Meanwhile, it would also be helpful for you to consult your medical professional effectively.

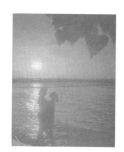

*E*jaculation is the most desirable, visible sign of orgasm for men. Mental aspect has played a major role in many occurrences of its disorders. However, some physical causes do exist.

24

Disorders of Ejaculation and Orgasm

While the problem with the ability to initiate, maintain, or sustain a penile erection is the most common cause for men to seek medical attention and help for their sexual difficulties, a few men may have some concern over their timing or feeling of ejaculation. Such a man may state that he came too fast, even before he could penetrate his wife or partner; this is called *premature ejaculation*. Or a man may say, "When I ejaculated, I felt it hurt or very painful inside."; this is *painful ejaculation*. Or at times, a man may say, "It took me for a long time or forever to get an ejaculation."; this may called *retarded ejaculation*.

Retrograde Ejaculation:

Normally, the direction of the spurts of ejaculation is coming forward and toward the end of your urethra (channel). This event is accomplished by "perfect" coordination between the contraction of the muscles at the immediate opening of the bladder (to close the bladder neck) and the relaxation of the muscles distal to the ejaculatory duct openings (to open up the sphincter) at the time of ejaculation. That is how it used to be.

However, if the normal closing ability of the muscles at the bladder neck is altered or reversed, retrograde ejaculation will occur. The common causes that impair the normal closing ability of bladder neck and lead to retrograde ejaculation are, **1.)** *a surgery or injury to the bladder neck,* **2.)** *a damage to the sympathetic nerves that control ejaculation,* **3.)** *an ingestion of the medications to block the transmission of sympathetic nerves for treating hypertension or psychotic disorders,* **4.)** *a spinal cord injury involving the sympathetic nerves to close the bladder neck at ejaculation,* and even **5.)** *a nerve damage from diabetes mellitus,* so-called *diabetic neuropathy.* Among all these, a surgery on the prostate, usually transurethral resection of the prostate (TURP), is the most common to be blamed because TURP, or its related procedure, is frequently performed for slow urination from an enlarged prostate after conservative treatment (usually with medication) failed. In fact, it is the expected consequence after this surgery that is usually done for the elderly. Despite retrograde ejaculation resulting from a reverse in the direction of ejaculatory flow, a pleasurable feeling from orgasm will still be present. For the details of an individual event and if any concern arises, please ask and discuss with your medical professionals.

To confirm the diagnosis of retrograde ejaculation, and if it is practically necessary, a microscopic examination of the voided urine after orgasm is needed. If the content of semen, usually sperms, is present, this diagnosis is correct. However, usually no treatment to reverse it is required because it usually occurs in the elderly who have no concern to raise more children.

At times, retrograde ejaculation may be confused with no ejaculation after any surgery to remove the seminal vesicles and/or completely block the ejaculatory ducts. The condition after radical prostatectomy is the most common cause for **no ejaculation** because this radical surgery for prostate cancer is so common in today's medical practice. In addition, it is worthwhile to know that this radical prostate removal may leave about one-third of the patients no presence of orgasm, one-third a reduced intensity of orgasm, and only about 20% no change in the quality of orgasm.

Premature Ejaculation:

What is the definition of premature ejaculation? Although the term, premature ejaculation itself seems quite explicit and it can be confusing to many people, it is necessary to search a definition from the perspectives of the patient and his partner. In this context, if a man ejaculates sooner than the time what he wants to in order to satisfy himself or sexual partner, this untimely early ejaculation is qualified to be called *premature ejaculation*. In other words, this man got frustrated because he was not able to make himself or sexual partner satisfied due to the premature occurrence of his ejaculation.

To understand the significance of premature ejaculation, it is helpful for men to know some facts of Nature in sex life. Notably, men need to know that most men will ejaculate after three to five minutes of regular vaginal penetration. In other words, under normal mental excitement and within a certain amount of friction between vaginal wall and the penis, a man's ejaculation will inevitably come no matter what. So, with this reality in mind, a man may be able to adjust and control his degree of mental excitement and the pace to accumulate the amount of friction between the vaginal wall and his penis in order to ejaculate timely and to satisfy himself and sexual partner. For controlling mental excitement, a man needs to be sure that his sexual intercourse is not conducted under undue stress such as in a hurry, with performance anxiety, or fear. As well, if direct foreplay is over done, the level of sexual excitement may advance too fast to control his ejaculation. Meanwhile, the pace of accumulating the needed amount of frictions between the vaginal wall and the penis can be adjusted by slowing the frequency of vaginal penetration and/or by adjusting the depth of vaginal penetration. All these measures are within the reach of our common sense to understand and practice. However, while a man is making an effort to adjust and work within his limit as just described, he should never ignore the pace of sexual excitement of his partner. To do so, please refer back to Parts II and III for details.

Out of curiosity, of course, you would like to know why a premature ejaculation does happen to you, especially when it just recently occurs. Many psychosocial difficulties in men or women, or both, including an extensive variety of mental complexes involving depression, anxiety, guilt, resentment, etc. have been blamed. However, the complexity of the subject is beyond the scope of this book. If a man fails to improve his control over the timing of ejaculation, he would need to see a qualified medical professional for advanced sexual counseling.

For treatment, in addition to the practice of self correction as just stated, probably in many your readings elsewhere, you may have noted a wide range of descriptions on many tips and hints to correct premature ejaculation; the common examples are the techniques of mental distraction, or the use of a condom, or the topical application of an agent, or an adjustment of the depth of vaginal penetration, or the practice of the famous Masters and Johnson method of the squeeze technique, etc. However, all the available measures are directed to moderate the degree, and pace, of mental and physical excitement at various levels of the nerve system.

For the details of using medications or applying various techniques, please consult with the qualified medical professionals. Nonetheless, most men with premature ejaculation can be corrected through self understanding and self improvement.

Painful Ejaculation:

Any discomfort, ache, or severe pain in or around a man's genital organs that appears at, or around, the time of ejaculation can be very distracting, unpleasant, and even frustrating. This event is not uncommon; it usually suggests some inflammatory or obstructive diseases in the internal genital organs such as the *prostate, seminal vesicles, vas deferens,* or *urethra.* The inflammatory process may be bacterial in origin, but nonbacterial is more common. For instance, a diagnosis of *prostatitis* has been very frequently used for the men with a symptom-complex of some discomfort in urination, urinary hesitancy, frequency, urgency, or discomfort in the area between the sac and the anus (*perineum*) without any bacterial evidence. Yet, unfortunately, many these men might have been treated with a long history of taking various antibiotics without improvement. Fortunately, a detailed history and a focused physical examination with a special attention to the beginning (onset), duration, and interval of pain as related with ejaculation, and an application of common sense by an experienced medical professional usually can define the cause and provide an appropriate treatment.

Besides, some conditions caused by cancerous diseases, or surgery, can result in an obstruction, or irritation, of the internal genital organs and cause painful ejaculation. Prostate cancer, or metastatic cancers from either elsewhere in the body or in the space between the rectum and the prostate and/or bladder, are the common examples. As stated, surgery to the prostate, or the vas deferens, or the scar formation inside the urethra may cause local pain at, or around, the time of ejaculation. However, such painful conditions after radical prostatectomy and vasectomy, and the occurrence of urethral stricture are fortunately not as common as it sounds to be.

To care and understand the details of painful ejaculation, it would be most desirable to see a urologist, but only the urologist who will follow the disciplined process of evaluation and management can do a real job for these patients. In reality, some urologists may just give the men with the above described symptom-complexes some antibiotics indiscriminately for the purpose of convenience. While many men with painful ejaculation can be cured, some may improve, a few may persist even under the care of the most disciplined urologists. As you know, there is a limit in medical care. Nonetheless, a good care for painful ejaculation can be available.

Retarded Ejaculation:

For a man with retarded ejaculation, he will experience a persistent difficulty in ejaculating, or a complete inability to ejaculate, although he has an adequate sexual desire, a proper sexual stimulation, and an erection This condition has been confused with the slow ejaculation that is related with normal aging change or frequent, untimely sexual intercourse. Common sense, and an understanding of the information described in Part III, will help a man solve the confusion and avoid unnecessary frustration. In general, it is not common, probably in less than 0.5% of men, although there is no good information about its real incidence.

However, the causes for retarded ejaculation may be organic or psychogenic. The organic causes may be drug-induced, or spinal cord-related, even diabetes mellitus, or any conditions that may affect the pathway for the input, or output, of sexual stimulation and information. And those of psychogenic causes may be related with anxiety, fear, a distorted thought about intercourse, or a conscious or subconscious distraction from the inside or the outside of the affected men. Some of them can be traced back to a traumatic event, which can eventually lead to a severe inhibition of ejaculation. Many may be so deeply seeded that an effort to solve it may prove to be very difficult. Fortunately, as stated, a real retarded ejaculation is not common.

To reveal the individual reality of the cause for retarded ejaculation and to explore the options of possible treatment, it would be beneficial and most reasonable to work and cooperate with your experienced medical professionals. Usually, a disciplined approach will be taken. If the cause is drug-related, a discontinuation, or adjustment, of the suspected drug may correct the problem. However, those related with deeply seeded psychogenic situations may be difficult to treat. However, if the practice for perfect sex fails to improve retarded ejaculation, you are advised to see an experienced medical professionals, usually a urologist first to rule an organic causes, and a psychologist or a psychiatrist to follow for timely sex counseling and treatment.

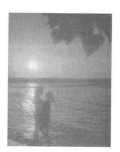

A summary is for quick reference. If there is any doubt, always look back on the details. If a doubt still exists, please consult with your caring, honest medical professionals.

25
A Summary of Causes and Treatment Options of Male Sexual Difficulties

This summary will give you a quick reference to the available options of treatment for male sexual difficulties. However, it is still mandatory to pay attention to the practice of those basic principles as described in Parts II and III. There is nothing magic in rehabilitating your sexual difficulties. We medical professionals will only fulfill our missions to make your sexual functions work for you as well, and as long, as possible. No matter what causes a man's sexual difficulties, the attitude and approach remain the same.

Among the treatment options, basic sex counseling (Level 1) as described in Section 19 is always the initial, first step of treatment and is required for any forms of male sexual difficulties. And penile implant is always considered as the last resort of treatment for erectile difficulties. The following table is not intended to complete an entire list of all the causes and treatments for all male sexual difficulties. Instead, it is intended only to use as a general reference guide. The details of medications and sequence of treatment may vary due to the individual need of patients as well as the "style and need" of the practice of individual medical professional.

Conditions or Causes	Treatment Options
1. Performance anxiety/fear 2. Isolated failure in erection	Basic or advanced sex counseling, occasionally medication, possible vacuum constriction device (VCD) or implant
3. Loss of desire (libido)	Basic or advanced sex counseling, medication of choice
4. Other psychosexual difficulties	Basic or advanced sex counseling
5. Other deviant sexual behaviors	Advanced long-term sex counseling
6. Arterial blockage	Basic sex counseling, optimize physical and mental states, sildenafil (Viagra) or other drugs, VCD, possible revascularization from trauma, penile implant as last resort
7. Leakage of penile veins	Basic sex counseling, VCD with medication of choice, selective ligation of penile veins, penile implant as last resort

Conditions or Causes cont.	**Treatment Options** cont.
8. Low male hormone (testosterone)	Testosterone supplement, preferably by intramuscular injection
9. High prolactin and pituitary tumor	Medication and/or surgery
10. After radical surgery for the cancer of prostate gland or rectal colon	Basic sex counseling, medication of choice and/or VCD, penile implant as last resort
11. Diabetes mellitus	Basic sex counseling, medication and/or device of choice, penile implant
12. Nerve injuries from spinal cord injuries, brain injuries or surgery	Basic sex counseling, medication and/or device of choice, penile implant
13. Drugs (prescribed or non-prescribed)	Basic sex counseling, discontinue or adjust dosage of drugs
14. After priapism	Basic sex counseling, medication or VCD of choice, penile implant
15. Penile deformity at birth or after surgery	Basic sex counseling, possible surgical reconstruction
16. Peyronie's disease	Basic sex counseling, medication of choice, less invasive surgery to correct undue curvature, penile implant

Conditions or Causes cont.	**Treatment Options** cont.
17. Premature ejaculation	Basic and advanced sex counseling, medication
18. No ejaculation	Basic sex counseling, reveal underlying cause and provide possible treatment
19. Retrograde ejaculation	Basic sex counseling, reveal consequence after prostate surgery or medication
20. Painful ejaculation	Basic sex counseling, treat inflammation or infection
21. Delayed ejaculation	Basic sex counseling for aging changes, advanced sexual counseling for refractory cases

Part V

●

A Brief on Potential Sexual Perversions

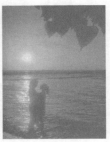

There is a thin line between normalcy and abnormality so that a dispute over any subject would never end. However, for contemporary general human value of life it is abnormal if the outcome of an act will bring about an adverse effect onto one's surroundings.

26
What are Abnormal Sexual Behaviors?

The discussion in prior sections was mainly applicable to the real life of the majority of people in society. It was not intended to be a set of rigid "rules or regulations" to exclude the minority of any nature in a society. As a urologist, I am not saying who is right or wrong. Instead, it is a part of my professional mission to explore a reasonable approach for people to pursue, and create, a better quality of life by helping them perfect their own sex life.

To further clarify, and intensify, the original intent of this book, it would be understandably useful to take some uncommon forms of sexual behaviors into consideration as a further discussion. People that desire to display deviant or abnormal sexual behaviors are potentially responsible for taking a risk to affect the overall balance, quality, and harmony of the real life of individuals, couples, and the society in which they live.

Under the governing freedoms of our Constitution, it is a true honor to observe the practice of people exercising their individual rights of free speech to verbally and openly express their opinion on any issue. With today's ever-expanding spirit of individualism, people and groups are becoming increasingly assertive as they demand "freedom" of expression in all forms. And to an extreme, over-assertion of rights may inevitably ignore, and overrun, their obligation; conflicts between the majority and the minority of interest groups occur all the time. For instances, the conflicts between pro-abortion and antiabortion groups have been a common scene throughout the United States in recent years. The heat of dispute on the issues of abortion does not stop at the level of verbal or written expression of different opinion. The extremists of anti-abortion push their level of expression to violence. Worst, they use killing people as their natural last mean to assert their rights and concerns over the issues of abortion. Similar situations for other interests have been happening from coast to coast as well.

Although there is a wide range of individual expression of sexual behaviors, they all serve a similar purpose in life: for procreation, for pleasure, for recreation, and so on. However, only certain kinds of variations in sexual behaviors are acceptable by an individual, a couple, or the majority of people in any given society. But in any relationship, there will always be individual need, limitations, and acceptances of certain forms of abnormal sexual behaviors. And for this reason, it would be insightful for a couple to actually sit down and negotiate their individual sexual needs.

If a person or a people "choose" to be the minority instead

of being part of the mainstream of society, they must also accept the consequences, and inconveniences, of their decision. For example, allow me to share something personal with you. I personally believe that there is a strong conflict of interest between making money for a living and decision-making when it comes to total patient care. To minimize and even avoid the feeling of such a conflict, I decided to quit my private medical practice and work for someone else. But by no means does anyone have to endure all the bitterness of being in a minority. Everyone has a choice and a need to resolve his or her personal wants, needs, and desires in a peaceful manner. In short, the expression by the majority in a given society should be considered as a normal aspect and determination of normality within a given society simply by the basic fact that "majority rules," but keep in mind, majorities also change from time to time.

What Forms of Sexual Behaviors are Considered to Be Abnormal?

This is a difficult question to answer. Being normal or abnormal is usually associated with the thoughts of being healthy or unhealthy, and is relative to the situation of the person, time, place, etc. There is a transitional gap between both ends. This gap may be viewed as the tolerance, or threshold, of an individual, or a couple, or a society. Normality and abnormality change within societies from time to time, person to person, couple to couple, society to society, culture to culture, and so on. Whatever "world of thought" predominates at the time becomes the norm... anything else would be considered abnormal to the accepted belief.

The expression of sexual behaviors is under the combined influences of hereditary, genetic, and various social factors in one's environment. For example, men holding hands and walking together is viewed as a sign of homosexuality in Western industrial countries while it is considered to be merely friendly behaviors in some other Cultures.

What is normal? It presents a condition or pattern that is possessed by the majority of people in a society. For example, in our society, most people will usually drive a car at a price that is compatible with their income. By doing so, they will be financially comfortable. That is *normal.* You may ask, "What does this example have something to do with a happy sex life?" Just wait and see.

Let us look at another scenario of life. For some reason, if a family is constantly spending more than its income can afford, this family sooner or later will have trouble balancing finances. This would be considered abnormal. Fortunately, most people budget their money and make timely adjustments in their cost of living expenditures whenever financial problems arise. Now, this would be considered normal behavior within the society. However, some people cannot make timely adjustments in their expenditures and must suffer the consequence from overspending. Such actions would then be considered abnormal "fiscal" responsibility.

In every society, people know that they need to wake up and take care of their daily routine chores and work for a living. They also need to sleep and rest for a good recovery from their mental and physical drainage during previous working and waking hours. This alternating repetitive cycles of life is an acceptable natural pattern. This is *normal.*

Some people have a wide "normal range" of variation, fluctuation, and scope in their mental and physical abilities.

That is why they may have a higher degree of durability and tolerance than others, especially during their youth. In spite of this blessed gift, the reserve of their mental and physical abilities will be drained, sooner or later, if they continuously engage in a living pattern of heavy work and less rest over an unreasonably extended time. Indeed, some people are very proud of what they can do in life because of their exceptional high tolerance or durability. However, if they over-stretch themselves to a level where they might feel that things are not right. In other words, they will eventually burn out. This is understandable. However, from the standpoint of working and living ability, it has become abnormal, which could directly influence one's own sexuality and that of their partner's.

To avoid any overindulgence in anything demands a need for moderation or balance in one's life. This coordinated thinking will bring a person to normality. To the very truth of life, if anything goes wrong, there is always a reason behind it. Unfortunately, a person's ego tends to obscure and deny the real reasons for overindulgence. Most of time, people tend to blame situational factors of time, place, and/ or someone else rather themselves. In our society, it has been especially true and inventive in imagining and creating an unlimited list of excuses for everything "wrong" (usually by legal and medical professionals). For example, there are many people who are really unacceptable and unruly in their behaviors. In order to excuse their legal responsibility for their wrongdoing, the thoughts of insanity and the suspicion of genetic defects are frequently orchestrated and presented by a joint effort of medical and legal professions to gain an undeserved public sympathy.

Now, let us look at some similar occurrences that might

influence someone's sex life. Traditional thinking has led our society to believe that sex life is a very personal, private matter. And no one else would question someone's lifestyles, particularly the matter of sex life. However, to some people, sexual overindulgence can be a common tendency in life under the pressure of desire to pursue sexual pleasure. Consequently, it may become problematic for them because of the over-drainage of their mental and physical reserves and the subsequent impairment in their ability of task or job performance. But people around them would not say a word to them without letting them feel being embarrassed or offended. For this reason, it would be wise for people to recognize what a "normal range" of sexual activity is.

Let us look at the sexual pattern of a gentleman at age 45. When he was 20 years old, let us assume, his refractory period (the time of inability to have sexual intercourse after an orgasm and ejaculation) was about 4-6 hours (if he just enjoyed sexual pleasure with intercourse without doing anything else.) In other words, he would maximally be able to have sexual intercourse 4 to 6 times over a period of 24 hours. Naturally, this would be an extreme for him. But, unfortunately, his wisdom fails to remind him timely that he is overextending himself and continues to desire and partake in sexual intercourse four to six times per day, as usual, even though he is now 45 years old. This is obviously an abnormal demand on himself. Eventually, he will fail.

At his present age, 45, his refractory period has slowly increased over the years. Now, let us assume it is about 20 to 30 hours. Based on this fact, his maximal ability to have intercourse is about once a day. If his pleasurable memory of sexual intercourse makes him insist to have intercourse more than once a day, apparently he is disobeying the natural laws of Nature, alternating work and recovery. Now, imagine what his real life could be. Because of his overindulgence, his job performance is impaired and he eventually loses his job. How can he then make a living? Now, he is in an "abnormal or diseased" condition. And what is the possible treatment that will bring him back to normality? Clearly, time and Nature are the best choice of care for him. And hopefully, in time, he will return to a more balanced path in life. But, in case he refuses to follow the suggested care, and he is no longer able to work, society will have to take care of him, and he becomes a burden upon society. However, he should ultimately be responsible for what he does although he may, as is usual in most people, blame someone, or something, else that caused this problem.

Through this direction of understanding, it is easy to sense what is considered to be normal (healthy) or abnormal (unhealthy) expressions of sexual behaviors. To be normal or abnormal is not solely reserved for individual accountability. Choice in life affects everyone and has far-reaching effects into any given society. If an individual's personal sexual preference changes in life, the change could have devastating effects on friends, family, and one's own sexual partner.

In summary, from personal and social standpoint, any sexual behaviors that fail to fulfill the goals of enriching the quality of life of involved individuals, couples, and society as a whole, are considered to be unhealthy, or even "abnormal".

What are the Commonly Mentioned Abnormal (or Unhealthy) Sexual Behaviors in Males and Females?

From the previous discussion, I assume that you have a reasonable understanding of what is meant by being normal (or healthy) or abnormal (or unhealthy) from a medical standpoint of view. Now, let us continue into what are the common types of abnormal (or unhealthy) sexual problems or disorders.

There are many special medical terms in psychology and psychiatry for sexually abnormal behaviors. They may not be familiar to many readers and even to some medical professionals that are not directly, and frequently, involved in the care of sexual difficulties. The reason for providing this list of sexual disorders is to allow the reader a general overview of the spectrum, or range, of problems from various and unusual sexual behaviors. It is also beneficial for anyone that may have a special interest to study the related subjects further.

According to the *Diagnostic and Statistical Manual-III* (DSM-III) of the American Psychiatric Association, the following sexual behaviors are considered to be abnormal (or unhealthy). These abnormal sexual behaviors can not only produce a significant undue effect on the offenders but can also inflict various degrees of harm to their victims.

Gender Identity Disorders:

The formation of a "normal" gender identity results from a satisfactory coordination and development between genetic coding and social, sexual orientation and preference of a person. However, in spite of genetic coding and guidance, the variations in the intensity of cultural beliefs, parental interactions, social exposure, etc. can lead to an imbalance in social, sexual orientation and preference. To the affected persons, such an adaptation in sexual orientation and preference is for the feeling of their own security but without knowing the undesirable impacts onto their surroundings that result from their social sexual behaviors.

- ### Gender Identity Disorders of Childhood, Adolescence or Adult Life:

During the process of development from childhood to adulthood, at times and more or less, a minor "crisis" of gender identity may temporarily surface in many persons. However, it usually self-correcting and may disappear in time with no significant adverse effect onto a person's later life. However, few may need medical help. And occasionally some may develop severe thought distortions about their gender identity.

A person with gender identity disorders has a feeling of discomfort or uneasiness about the appearance of their external genital organ. Their sexual behaviors are generally associated with those of the opposite sex. *Therefore, any children or adults with these features should be (if they are troubled) counseled into seeking the help of a medical professional, usually in the field of psychology or psychiatry because such persons have severe difficulty in sexual preference and orientation*. The detail of evaluation and care for them is certainly beyond the scope of this book. Nevertheless, it is useful for anyone to have at least a general knowledge about the problem from these poor sexual adjustments. And a timely medical attention and care from psychologists or psychiatrists may be obtained to minimize the occurrence of the difficulty from gender identity disorders.

- ### Transsexualism:

A person with transsexualism feels an overwhelming uneasiness with their own sexual appearance and may have a constant desire to get rid of their own external genital organs in order to become a member of the opposite sex. It is a condition of a fully blown extreme of gender identity disorders.

For the purpose of making a diagnosis, such a mental condition needs to persist for more than two years. It is not associated with schizophrenia. It is not a common urological disorder although it is sometimes observed in major medical centers. The patient usually requests urological/surgical procedures to change the external appearance of their sexual organs to that of the opposite sex in addition to the use of sexual hormone of opposite sex. Before considering, and deciding, on a procedure to convert the appearance of their sexual organs to those of opposite sex, a joint consultation between patient, psychiatrist, and an experienced urologist is needed. In other words, the whole care for the patients with transsexualism is a major multidisciplinary task.

Paraphilias:

"Para" usually implies "resembling or similar to." "Philia" means an abnormal attraction to something. The word, paraphilia means having a tendency to love something in an abnormal way. It is more or less close to a feeling of perversion. It is considered to be abnormal (unhealthy) as compared to the normal standard pattern of sexual behaviors.

For a person with paraphilia, erotic sexual arousal and gratification is quite different from that of the normal standard majority of people. The main interests of a paraphilia is their persistence and repetition to be sexually aroused by fantasies, commonly of an unusual nature. They tend to use non-human objects for their sexual arousal. Paraphilias are aroused through sexual activities with humans involving a real or simulated suffering or humiliation, as well as, with non-consenting partners. With this in mind, it would be easy to know the following terms.

• *Fetishism*

It indicates a person's preference to exclusively use some type of nonliving object to achieve their sexual arousal and gratification. An article of clothing is the most common fetish. A minor degree of this type of behavior is not necessarily deemed to be "abnormal." To a certain degree, most of us are somewhat fetishistic. If the degree of this behavior becomes acute and affects one's normal sexual relationship, the condition will be obviously abnormal and unhealthy. Under this condition, such people tend to avoid a normal sexual relationship. The real goal of pure fetishism is masturbation, not sexual contact. The fetishists use nonliving sexual objects to replace human relationship.

• *Transvestism*

Individuals of transvestism like to cross-dress to achieve sexual stimulation. This condition may not have a significant problem for maintaining a reasonably normal and happy sexual relationship as long as the partner is understanding and cooperative. However, there may be an emotional conflict if an individual senses anxiety, depression, shame, and/or guilt. These people also tend to have other types of paraphilias, most commonly fetishism.

• *Zoophilia*

"Zoo" means animals. Zoophilias prefer to have sexual stimulation and arousal through the act or fantasy of engaging in sexual activities with animals. It is a very rare disorder.

• *Pedophilia*

It is a most commonly reported sexual offense in our society. It is an abnormal condition that exists in certain individuals that compel themselves to have and desire sexual relationship with children, related or unrelated. This abnormal condition seems to be found more in males than in females by a ratio of 2:1. When an incident such as this occurs within the immediate family, it is known as incest.

• *Exhibitionism*

It describes a condition of repetitively exposing a person's genital organs to an unsuspecting stranger for producing sexual stimulation and excitement in themselves. The more surprised or shocked the victims respond, the more the sexual excitement the offenders will have. Offenders are usually males and their victims are females. Occasionally, though, females may be the offenders also.

• *Voyeurism*

A person displaying voyeurism desires to experience sexual arousal through repetitive acts of viewing an unsuspecting person (usually a woman) who is in the process of disrobing, being naked, or engaging in sexual activities. At times, they may have orgasm, usually, through masturbation, which may occur during their voyeuristic activities. Pornography is essentially a form of voyeurism. They avoid physical sexual contacts.

• *Sexual Masochism*

A person that exhibits sexual masochism will intentionally participate in activities in which are physically harmful or threatening to their lives in order to generate their sexual excitement. Frequently, they also enjoy sexual excitement by being humiliated, bound, beaten or otherwise made to suffer.

• *Sexual sadism*

It is a form of producing sexual excitement and orgasm by inflicting physical or psychological suffering on a sexual partner. Rape, torture, and murder are the extreme forms of sexual sadism.

• *Coprophilia*

It is used to describe a love of feces (stool) through a rare nonstandard sexual behavior.

• *Frotteurism*

People with this condition like to rub against an unsuspecting stranger in order to produce sexual excitement.

• *Klismaphilia*

Individuals with this condition sexually stimulate and excite themselves through self-inducement (autoerotism) of enemas.

• *Mysophilia*

It is a description for a person that likes to experience sexual excitement in a filthy environment.

• *Necrophilia*

In a person with necrophilia, sexual excitement is produced through sexual activity with a dead body.

• *Telephone scatologia*

This is to describe an obsessive act to make an obscene telephone call to a stranger for sexual stimulation. It is very common in today's society.

• *Urophilia*

A person with urophilia is sexually stimulated when they urinate (void) onto another person that may or may not a willing participant.

Psychosexual Dysfunctions

This is a grouping of sexual difficulties that mainly influence the strength of sexual desire and the ability of sexual excitement, orgasm and pleasure. The common conditions in men are inhibited sexual desire, sexual excitement, orgasm, premature ejaculation, and so on. Those for females are inhibited sexual desire, sexual excitement, orgasm, some forms of painful sexual intercourse, and spasm of muscles around the vagina, and others.

Other Psychosexual Disorders

A man who desires to convert to a heterosexual orientation after a period of a stressful homosexual relationship would be an example. All of these abnormalities involve a higher level of psychological difficulties that would require a skillful psychological or psychiatric care by the medical professionals in these special fields.

I hope there is no confusion over these terms. As mentioned before, the information provided is intended to give the reader a general impression about the complications and aspects of deviant sexual behaviors in a given society.

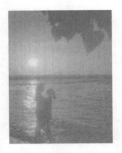

A bnormality disturbs the harmony and graciousness of normality. And vice versa. Only a clear visualization of convincing benefits from the value of normality can possibly bring the "victims" of abnormality back to the camp of normality.

27
Social Implication of Abnormal Sexual Behaviors?

Although most people enjoy their sex life with a pattern of normal or healthy forms of sexual expression, few prefer to reveal their sexual expressions dramatically different from that of the majority of people. Of course, as a rule, these few also want to feel their sexual security despite the contents of their sexual revelation are not well perceived and accepted by most people. Nonetheless, their presence is the- reality of social life. We can not get rid of them but we may be able to do something about it and to help these few.

What is the social implication of these so-called deviated abnormal or unhealthy sexual behaviors? All of these deviant behaviors are not considered to be the normal standard pattern of sexual behaviors. They all use the unusual means to generate sexual stimulation and excitement at the expense of someone's pleasure, suffering, non-consent, or even humiliation. They are not accepted nor appreciated by the majority of people. Also, they tend to be repetitive and obsessive in nature. The worst example is sexually related serial killer, such as James Damler.

For the harmony of a society and the betterment of general public health, these sexual behaviors are considered abnormal or unhealthy by the public and need to be contained and curbed. There is a deep public resentment toward these people that display (openly) deviated sexual behaviors. At times, their behaviors cross the line and become criminal offenses. What is needed in this society is a program from which the offenders of this nature may receive a timely support and help. Proper medical attention will allow some of these people to receive a needed help that will allow them to still dearly need, to convert their abnormal sexual behaviors to the main stream of normality.

If society opens its heart and really looks into the origin and issue of an offender's sexual behaviors, *the root of their current expression of unhealthy sexual behaviors can almost always be traced back to their early upbringing.* Therefore, it is very important for the general public to be reasonably aware of the close relationships between their current sexual behaviors and what they had seen, heard, touched, smelled, and experienced as a child. And, through a similar public awareness that has been used on the programs for various cancer diseases, more people will be alerted to the complications and aspects of abnormal sexual behaviors. More people will be able to sense and pay close attention to the early signs of such a possible development and occurrence of these abnormal sexual behaviors in their own family. Subsequently, it would become easier for more and more people to know what is normal or abnormal for sexual behaviors. Such public awareness will bring the issue of abnormal sexual behaviors to the forefront of public knowledge and news instead of dodging and ignoring them when they occur. Only through a positive and constructive attitude toward such issues, the seriousness of the problem will be fully recognized and diffused in a timely fashion within our society. Hopefully, abnormal sexual behaviors will be recognized early enough in a child and not be allowed to fully develop later in their adult life. Later development will only complicate matters and handicap the affected persons in their developing a normal relationship and/or healthy behavior in the future.

Therefore, the more public awareness of such events (complicated "unacceptable" sexual behaviors), the more effective these unhealthy sexual behaviors can be diffused, minimized, and even avoided. I hope there will be more parents and adults that would be willing to participate and activate their interest in knowing more about the existence and effects of unhealthy sexual behaviors. By helping our younger generation understand what "normal and acceptable" sexual behaviors are in a society, we will, as a society, eventually see the rate of unhealthy behaviors begin to decrease.

Today, abnormal sexual behaviors have been reported by all forms of news media as a form of social or national soap opera. There was a time in America when the majority of society would have been upset, angry, disappointed, and would have thoroughly condemned these acts. But now, there seems to be an increasing tolerance for such behaviors. Experts in this field explain that many people are no longer shocked by such behavior of such events. And in deed, many people today view the revealing of these unhealthy sexual acts as if they are watching an soap opera. As a nation, as a people, and as individuals, it must be noted that when any abnormal behavior is tolerated by any society, it will eventually become accepted by the society; and once it is accepted, it becomes a commonplace. Then, the perpetrators will be happier as they watch a helpless society falter in discussion and reaction. These reactions would probably make them even more intensely interested in making more trouble to satisfy themselves.

In order to curb these unhealthy behaviors in society effectively, people and government need to do more than just what current social policies can offer. Society needs to step up the publicity and educate the general public, schools and individuals to face and discuss these growing issues. Hopefully, educational efforts will generate a preventive effect to minimize the occurrence of these unhealthy sexual behaviors in a foreseeable future.

Most human beings are born with and basically equipped with five natural senses: hearing, seeing, smelling, touching, and tasting. Along with these natural senses, humans are also able to reason and think, integrating incoming information through a complex thought process. And because of the existence of hereditary and genetic factors, there is a wide range of learning differences among most humans, which, of course, cannot be changed or modified. However, the whole learning process first begins in the early years of the family unit and then continues later in society. There are also many learning variables throughout an individual's life that are capable of changing or altering one's belief, opinion, acceptance, and tolerance of certain ideals and convictions such as morals, religion, sex, etc. And regardless of age, one's individual mental and physical activities are constantly changing and modifying. But, in spite of this, there is a general direction that all humans seem to follow as they age, they seem to become more and more selective and ever restrictive in their beliefs, opinions, acceptances, and tolerances as time goes by.

In general, we are not really that different from wild animals. Relying on all five senses plus the integrating ability, we are able to feel, integrate, and react for survival, just like any other animal. And like all other newborn animals, human newborns are able to feel the sense of hunger, cry for food, move around, touch, smell the odor of their mother, feel the softness of their mother's breast, and open their mouth to suckle. And all newborns can do this without seeing, these inborn senses are a newborn's primitive instincts for survival.

Do all humans use these primitive instincts the same way? Of course, not. But through the process of parental nurturing, and later by the addition of various social activities, including schooling, the range of sensitivity and specificity is slowly developed. We become increasingly selective as we age, eventually, the patterns of sensing and integrating slowly develop and evolve into individual differences. That is why all humans are basically the same, and yet, so distinctly different in many ways.

Yet, humans are still able to live together peacefully through a constantly changing and adjusting process of mental and physical behaviors. Due to the changing environments, change has to happen in order for species to survive and feel safe. If the comfort point of sensing, integrating, changing, and adjusting is not in balance, an individual would have to act by doing something to reach another level of comfort and peace. The level of comfort and peace is quite different from individual to individual. However, the pattern of most comfort points in humans is predictable and acceptable by the majority of people. But there are some people at the extreme ends of comfort and peace, and these exceptions are considered abnormal and are not accepted by the majority of people. Therefore, as duly noted, humans are essentially born free and equal, but it is the early nurturing and learning process that influence and determine differences.

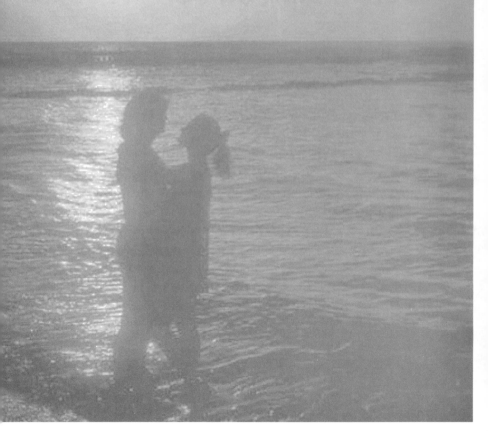

Part VI
●
Conclusion and General Advise

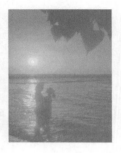

A t the end of a journey, we all like to look back at what we have gained through it. While the details of a journey may not be dearly remembered, its spirit and concept cannot be forgotten and becomes your wisdom.

28
Conclusion on Perfect Sex

Now, it is the time for us to wrap up what we have explored together in the search for perfect sex life. In the most primitive sense of human sexuality, sex is for **procreation**, which is much like that for any biological body.

However, from the points of view of immediate and remote effects of human sexuality, sex life is **the centerpiece of attention of our daily living as well as the non-spoken bonding power of family and society.**

In our contemporary sense, the content of sexuality may be viewed as a vibrant form of **relaxation, a mini-vacation, and/or a recreation of daily life** while it is used in a constructive, gracious, and dignitary way. In essence, sexuality has its own unique precious value and beauty for individuals and societies as described in Section 8, *Social Impact of Sex Life.*

Therefore, undoubtedly, sex life is **the most commonly available, natural resource** for every human being to explore and use.

For the benefits of our next generation, the value and beauty of sex life could be **the most blessed, treasured gift from God that we should preserve, enhance, and pass on**; it is much more than those that money can buy. To accomplish that, **all responsible fulfilling adults should act as a role model of perfect sex.**

For its daily function, the beauty and value of sex life could be used **as a tool of enhancing mutual quality of life.** However, in its operation toward perfect sex, we should **never use the need for sexual pleasure as a tool of leverage for dispute or negotiation.** If you do, the true inner relationship of a couple will surely deteriorate. And the pursuit of perfect sex would be impossible.

Because of the tremendous visible, and invisible, power and beauty of sex, every human being should make an effort to explore it to the extreme of achieving perfection as artists do. A perfect sex life can be viewed, and accomplished, as **a living work of art**. Therefore, pursuing perfection with the principles and methods as described in this book can make your fulfillment of "perfect sex" a reality.

While sex life is a personal matter, due to its "unlimited" enormous effects to a society, **as a nation**, we should **devote more time and money to conduct more research for promoting the concept and practice of perfect sex**. Use the real visualization of the beauty and value of sex life to attract more people and couples to practice perfect sex, not by governmental rules and regulations. To deliver the result of the findings, we should emphasize the understanding and practice with common sense and minimize the sacredness of a specialty that is beyond the reach of the public.

S exual pleasure is fun to enjoy. But safety and quality of life should come first.

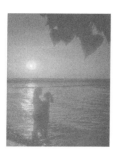

29
General Advice for Realistic, Safe Sex Life

Technically, and realistically, the performance of sex should be a constant part of daily life, although the act of sexual intercourse has been commonly isolated and viewed by many people as the sole part of sex life. In fact, it is not, but is the emotional and physical peak of total sexual performance. For easy understanding and good preparation to perform, it is useful to consider sexual intercourse as a job performance, which requires an adequacy of mental and physical preparation in order to do it well. Therefore, the appropriateness of indirect foreplay, direct foreplay, resolution, and recovery is essential and plays an indispensable role of mental and physical preparation and readiness.

To have an adequate mental comfort to perform, you need to be sure that you are free of anxiety and free of fear from personal, social, financial, and professional pressures. While to be completely free from these pressures is impossible, at least all the pressures of realistic daily life have to be reasonably contained under the level that is tolerable to a person. Without a relaxing and confident mind, quality of performance will be impaired in spite of a good physical condition. Therefore, it is wise to honestly review the status of personal, social, financial, and professional adequacy and make a sensible and realistic adjustment accordingly and timely. In an absolute sense, a person should be responsible for any inadequacy of her/his life; the affected person is the real, and only one, who can rescue herself/himself. Fortunately, especially in America, there are a lot of opportunities and resources around for any interested person to take advantage of it. We *in America* are truly in a lucky world.

To assure a physical fitness to act, within the reach of understanding and imagination, she/he needs to possess an affordable physical reserve to act out at the level that the body can tolerate without over-exertion. To optimally maximize physical affordability, it is reasonable to start out with good dietary habits. To consume any edibles in moderation and balance should be the beginning point *of dietary habits.* So doing, a person will most likely live under a balanced nutritional status. In addition, it is also essential to have an adequate amount of physical exercise; minimally, it is very advisable to make sure that all the joints of the body move within a tolerable limit (range of motion). As to the intensity of exercise, it should depend on an individual's realistic tolerance and durability. In general, it is a good idea to honestly listen to what the body signals. For any doubts of one's own body, please consult a medical professional. Such a physical maintenance should be a constant part of daily life.

For anyone with certain established chronic diseases such as diabetes mellitus, ischemic heart disease, kidney failure, liver failure, lung failure, etc., they are seriously advised to cooperatively follow the advice of medical professionals. As previously stated, a medical professional is a medical, artistic scientist that can help your body work as well, and as long, as possible.

With the need for proper mental and physical preparation and readiness in mind (and practice), a person will surely have the best possible condition to enjoy the peaked pleasure of orgasm from their ultimate sexual intimacy.

However, at closing, for someone with marginal physical ability, such as those of high age and/or with ischemic heart disease, I highly advise them to review, and follow, the following:

- Maintain and sustain an optimal condition of your mental comfort to perform and physical fitness to act.
- Quit smoking if you are a smoker.
- Do not have intercourse with a full stomach after a big meal.
- Do not have intercourse while you are intoxicated and/or after heavy drinking.
- Do not have intercourse when you are physically and mentally tired.
- Do not have intercourse when you have to do it in a hurry.
- Do not have intercourse whenever you are not comfortable with someone around the house.
- Find a mutual agreeable time, place, and mood to have intercourse.

- Sexual intercourse is for pleasure, yours and your sexual partner's, and not just to please sexual partner or you alone.

As you can see, all these precautions and efforts can make your overall mental and physical condition at its best. In other words. I like to see you make a best use out of your mental and physical abilities.

Finally, I would like to express my appreciation and thanks for your patience and effort in reading this book. Here, also, goes my sincere respect towards your good intention and effort to perfect the contents of your sex life. I hope your quality of life will be enhanced as well as your sexual partner. I further hope that the value, respect, beauty, and power of your sex life can be recognized, glorified, and passed onto our following generations to come endlessly.

Some Organizations to contact
(if you need more information)

American Foundation for Urologic Disease (AFUD)
300 West Pratt Street, Suite 401
Baltimore, MD 21201 -2463
410-727-2908 or 1-800-242-2383

Impotence Institute of America (IIA)
10400 Little Patuxent Parkway, Suite 485
Columbia, MD 21044-3502
1-800-669-1603

National Kidney and Urologic Diseases Information Clearinghouse
3 Information Way (attention: UP)
Bethesda, MD 20892-3580
301 -654-4415

American Association of Sex Educators, Counselors & Therapists (A.A.S.E.C.T.)
PO Box 238
Mt Vernon, IA 52314

Bibliography

1. Sexual Problems in Medical Practice,
   from American Medical Association, 1981.

2. Sexual Medicine and Counseling in Office Practice,
   first edition, by D. J. Munjack, M.D. and L. J. Oziel, M.D.,
   1980, from Little, Brown and Company.

3. Sex for Dummies, by Dr. Ruth K. Westheimer, 1995,
   from IDG Books Worldwide, Inc.

4. Evaluation and Treatment of Erectile Dysfunction, a Process of Care Model, from the University of Medicine and
   Dentistry of New Jersey, Robert Wood Johnson Medical
   School.

5. Sexual Nutrition, by Dr. Morton Walker from Avery Publishing Group, 1994

6. Sex for Beginners, by Errol Selkirk, from Writer and Readers Publishing, Inc., 1994